Responding to Problem Behavior in Schools

The Guilford Practical Intervention in the Schools Series

Kenneth W. Merrell, Series Editor

Helping Students Overcome Depression and Anxiety: A Practical Guide
Kenneth W. Merrell

Emotional and Behavioral Problems of Young Children:
Effective Interventions in the Preschool and Kindergarten Years
Gretchen A. Gimpel and Melissa L. Holland

Conducting School-Based Functional Behavioral Assessments:
A Practitioner's Guide
T. Steuart Watson and Mark W. Steege

Executive Skills in Children and Adolescents:
A Practical Guide to Assessment and Intervention
Peg Dawson and Richard Guare

Responding to Problem Behavior in Schools:
The Behavior Education Program
Deanne A. Crone, Robert H. Horner, and Leanne S. Hawken

Responding to Problem Behavior in Schools

The Behavior Education Program

DEANNE A. CRONE
ROBERT H. HORNER
LEANNE S. HAWKEN

THE GUILFORD PRESS
New York   London

© 2004 The Guilford Press
A Division of Guilford Publications, Inc.
72 Spring Street, New York, NY 10012
www.guilford.com

Printed in Canada

This book is printed on acid-free paper.

Last digit is print number: 9 8 7 6 5 4 3 2 1

Library of Congress Cataloging-in-Publication Data

Crone, Deanne A.
  Responding to problem behavior in schools : the behavior education
program / Deanne A. Crone, Robert H. Horner, Leanne S. Hawken.
        p. cm.
  Includes bibliographical references.
  ISBN 1-57230-940-7 (alk. paper)
  1. Behavior modification—United States. 2. School psychology—United
States. 3. Problem children—Education—United States. I. Horner,
Robert H. II. Hawken, Leanne S. III. Title.
  LB1060.2.C76 2004
    370.15′3—dc22   2003014174

About the Authors

Deanne A. Crone, PhD, is Assistant Professor of School Psychology at the University of Oregon. She has directed several research and training grants addressing behavior disorders, positive behavior support, and functional behavioral assessment. Dr. Crone has conducted extensive training in functional behavioral assessment and positive behavior support with teachers, paraprofessionals, principals, and directors of special education.

Robert H. Horner, PhD, is Professor of Special Education at the University of Oregon. He codirects several major research and technical assistance projects addressing positive behavior support. Dr. Horner also has coauthored research assessing the Behavior Education Program approach to behavior support.

Leanne S. Hawken, PhD, is Assistant Professor in the Special Education Program at the University of Utah. She has assisted schools in implementing the Behavior Education Program at both the elementary and middle school levels, and has conducted research studies to evaluate its effectiveness. Dr. Hawken's main research focus is positive behavior support, including school-wide behavior support, targeted interventions for at-risk students, and functional assessment/behavior support planning for students engaging in severe problem behavior.

Acknowledgments

We extend appreciation and credit to the faculty, staff, and students of Fern Ridge Middle School, Meadowview Elementary School, Bohemia Elementary School, Bethel School District, and Tigard–Tualatin School District for their innovations, suggestions, implementation efforts, and encouragement in the development of this book. We would also like to thank Rob March for his contributions to the initial research on the Behavior Education Program. A special thank you to Claudia Vincent for her tireless efforts and organization in the final stages of putting together the manuscript for this and other publications. Her assistance is always invaluable.

Contents

1

Introduction to the
Behavior Education Program

WHAT IS THE PURPOSE OF THE BOOK?

The purpose of this book is to describe a targeted system of positive behavior support called the Behavior Education Program (BEP): what it is, how it works, who can benefit from it, and how it is implemented in a school. The goal of the book is to provide the reader with the rationale, procedures, and tools to (1) determine if a BEP system is appropriate for your school, and (2) implement a variation of the BEP that fits the needs of your school.

The BEP is intended to be one part of the larger behavior support effort in a school. Schools that have effective and complete systems of positive behavior support in place address three levels of behavioral need:

1. All students must be taught the schoolwide rules and expectations.
2. At-risk students must have a system for reducing the risk that behavior will become worse over time.
3. Students with serious problem behavior must receive intensive, individualized behavior support.

The BEP addresses the second level of behavioral need. (For resources on the first and third levels of behavioral need, refer to the Resources section at the end of this chapter.) The BEP targets students who demonstrate persistent, but not dangerous, patterns of problem behavior. These are students who do not respond well to school-wide behavioral expectations. These are *not* students who require comprehensive, individualized interventions. The BEP should improve the overall efficiency of the school-wide procedures, while reducing the number of individualized interventions that are needed.

Resources in schools are dwindling. At the same time, schools are expected to do more to support students. This book provides teachers, administrators, school psychologists, and other school personnel with the tools to implement an *efficient* and *cost-effective* system of positive behavior support in their schools. The book details the logic, procedures, administrative systems, and forms needed to build a BEP system. Tools for ongoing evaluation and improvement of the system also are provided. A list of acronyms and definitions appears in Appendix A for a quick review of terms, as needed.

WHAT IS THE BEP?

The BEP is a school-based program for providing daily support and monitoring for students who are at risk for developing serious or chronic problem behavior. Students who fail to respond to school-wide approaches and who acquire several disciplinary referrals per year may benefit from a targeted group intervention like the BEP. It is based on a daily check-in/check-out system that provides the student with immediate feedback on his or her behavior (via teacher rating on a Daily Progress Report [DPR]) and increased positive adult attention. Expectations are clearly defined, and students are given both immediate and delayed reinforcement for meeting behavioral expectations. To increase home–school collaboration, a copy of the DPR is sent home to be signed by the parents or caregivers and brought back the next school day. A critical feature of the BEP is the use of data to evaluate its effectiveness in changing student behavior. Points earned on the DPR are graphed, and decisions are made weekly by the school's Behavior Support Team to either continue, modify, or fade the BEP intervention.

The BEP incorporates several core principles of positive behavior support, including (1) clearly defined expectations, (2) instruction on appropriate social skills, (3) increased positive reinforcement for following expectations, (4) contingent consequences for problem behavior, (5) increased positive contact with an adult in the school, (6) improved opportunities for self-management, and (7) increased home–school collaboration.

The BEP goes beyond its impact on a single student. It provides the school with a proactive, preventive response to serious problem behavior. In addition, the BEP intervention enhances communication among teachers, improves school climate, increases consistency among staff, and helps teachers to feel supported.

HOW IS THE BEP EFFICIENT AND COST-EFFECTIVE?

The BEP is continuously available, can be implemented within 3 days of identifying a problem, and typically requires no more than 5–10 minutes per teacher per day. Additional coordination time is required, but the key point is that this system can be used by all teachers and staff in a school, with low time demands. All staff are trained to implement the BEP intervention, which is continuously available for students who need additional positive behavior support. Unlike intensive, individualized interventions (i.e., those requiring a functional behavioral assessment and an extensive behavior support plan), no lengthy assessment process is conducted prior to the student receiving BEP support. The goal is for the student to be identified and receive support within 3 school days. Personnel time required to implement the intervention is minimal (see Chapter 5 for resource and time requirements), and many students (20–30) can be supported on the system at the same time.

WHY ARE TARGETED INTERVENTIONS LIKE THE BEP NECESSARY?

Most schools do not have the time or resources to provide comprehensive individualized behavior support for *all* students who need varying levels of extra support. For example, in a school with a population of 500 students, it is estimated that approximately 15–20%, or 75–100 students, will need more support than what school-wide prevention efforts provide. Conducting intensive, individualized interventions with all of these students would be timely and would tax school resources. Many students will respond to simple intervention strategies, like the BEP, that are less time-intensive and more cost-efficient to implement.

Implementing the BEP system in your school does not replace the need for intensive, individualized interventions. There will be students for whom the BEP will not be adequate to produce significant reductions in problem behavior. For those students, a functional behavioral assessment should be conducted, and data from the assessment should be used to develop an individualized behavior support plan. (For more information on intensive positive behavior support, see Crone & Horner, 2003.)

WHICH SCHOOLS SHOULD CONSIDER IMPLEMENTING THE BEP?

Schools that have a school-wide system of positive behavior support (Lewis & Sugai, 1999; Sugai & Horner, 2002) in place and that still have 10 or more students needing extra support should consider implementing the BEP. A school-wide system of positive behavior support clarifies expectations both for students and staff and also reduces the overall number of students who are engaging in problem behavior. If there are fewer than 10 students who engage in problem behavior, a school may be able to simply implement individualized behavior supports for each of them, rather than invest in the BEP.

Although the BEP is cost-efficient and requires very low effort by staff to implement, the commitment of *all* staff members and the support of the building administrator are crucial to the success of the program. Administrator support includes the allocation of personnel time and resources to implementation and ongoing evaluation of the intervention. Chapter 5 details the steps necessary to get the BEP started in your school and includes a self-assessment checklist to determine readiness for implementing the intervention system.

IF MY SCHOOL IS ALREADY IMPLEMENTING A SYSTEM LIKE THE BEP FOR AT-RISK STUDENTS, WILL I STILL BENEFIT FROM READING THIS BOOK?

Yes! This book may help you to make your BEP-type of system more efficient, or help you impose an organizing structure that you may currently lack. In Chapter 6, we discuss adaptations and elaborations of the BEP system that may help you identify effective modifications to be used when the basic BEP is inadequate for a particular student.

If your targeted intervention system is being implemented well, you are probably seeing a decrease in the number of students who need intensive behavior interventions. Many schools have a program(s) in place to support students who have difficulty meeting academic and behavioral expectations. Often, however, students are placed into these programs without attention to the reason behind the student's problem behavior. *Is the curriculum material too difficult for the student? Does the student act out to get a reaction from his peers? Does the student like staying in from recess and getting the one-to-one adult attention when she hasn't finished her class work?*

This book describes a brief assessment process to help school personnel think "functionally" about problem behavior, that is, to determine the reason for a student's problem behavior. If a student repeatedly engages in a problem behavior, a pattern will likely emerge. These patterns of behavior can be manipulated to decrease inappropriate behavior while increasing desired behavior. This brief assessment and intervention process is discussed in Chapter 6.

RESOURCES

Building School-Wide Systems of Positive Behavior Support

Bear, G. G. (1990). Best practices in school discipline. In A. Thomas & J. Grimes (Eds.), *Best practices in school psychology–II* (pp. 649–663). Washington, DC: National Association of School Psychologists.

Colvin, G., Kameenui, E. J., & Sugai, G. (1993). School-wide and classroom management: Reconceptualizing the integration and management of students with behavior problems in general education. *Education and Treatment of Children, 16*, 361–381.

Colvin, G., Sugai, G., Good, R. H., III, & Lee, Y. (1997). Using active supervision and precorrection to improve transition behaviors in an elementary school. *School Psychology Quarterly, 12*, 344–363.

Gottfredson, D. C., Gottfredson, G. D., & Skroban, S. (1996). A multimodel school based prevention demonstration. *Journal of Adolescent Research, 11*, 97–115.

Gottfredson, D. C., Karweit, N. L., & Gottfredson, G. D. (1989). *Reducing disorderly behavior in middle schools* (Report No. 47). Baltimore, MD: John Hopkins University, Center of Research on Elementary and Middle Schools.

Hyman, I., Flanagan, D., & Smith, K. (1982). Discipline in the schools. In C. R. Reynolds & T. B. Gutkin (Eds.), *The handbook of school psychology* (pp. 454–480). New York: Wiley.

Kazdin, A. E. (1982). Applying behavioral principles in the schools. In C. R. Reynolds & T. B. Gutkin (Eds.), *The handbook of school psychology* (pp. 501–529). New York: Wiley.

Knoff, H. M. (1985). Best practices in dealing with discipline referrals. In A. Thomas & J. Grimes

(Eds.), *Best practices in school psychology* (pp. 251–262). Washington, DC: National Association of School Psychologists.

Lewis, T. J., & Sugai, G. (1999). Effective behavior support: A systems approach to proactive school-wide management. *Focus on Exceptional Children, 31*(6), 1–24.

Lewis-Palmer, T., Sugai, G., & Larson, S. (1999). Using data to guide decisions about program implementation and effectiveness. *Effective School Practices, 17*(4), 47–53.

Mayer, G. R., Butterworth, T., Nafpaktitis, M., & Sulzer-Azaroff, B. (1983). Preventing school vandalism and improving discipline: A three year study. *Journal of Applied Behavior Analysis, 16,* 355–369.

Sugai, G., & Horner, R. H. (1999). Discipline and behavioral support: Preferred processes and practices. *Effective School Practices, 17*(4), 10–22.

Sulzer-Azaroff, B., & Mayer, G. R. (1994). *Achieving educational excellence: Behavior analysis for achieving classroom and schoolwide behavior change.* San Marcos, CA: Western Image.

Taylor-Greene, S., Brown, D., Nelson, L., Longton, J., Gassman, T., Cohen, J., Swartz, J., Horner, R. H., Sugai, G., & Hall, S. (1997). School-wide behavioral support: Starting the year off right. *Journal of Behavioral Education, 7,* 99–112.

Todd, A. W., Horner, R. H., Sugai, G., & Sprague, J. R. (1999). Effective behavior support: Strengthening school-wide systems through a team-based approach. *Effective School Practices, 17*(4), 23–27.

Building Individualized Behavior Support

Crone, D. A., & Horner, R. H. (2003). *Building positive behavior support systems in schools: Functional behavioral assessment.* New York: Guilford Press.

Fad, K. M., Patton, J. R., & Polloway, E. A. (1998). *Behavioral intervention planning.* Austin, TX: Pro-Ed.

Horner, R. H., Sugai, G., Todd, A. W., & Lewis-Palmer, T. (1999–2000). Elements of behavior support plans: A technical brief. *Exceptionality, 8*(3), 205–215.

Repp, A. C., & Horner, R. H. (Eds.). (1999). *Functional analysis of problem behavior: From effective assessment to effective support.* Belmont, CA: Wadsworth.

2

The Context for Positive Behavior Support in Schools

Schools face a growing challenge in meeting both the instructional and behavioral needs of all students. Students today are diverse and present educators with a unique set of challenges (e.g., English as second language, low socioeconomic status, significant learning and behavioral needs) (Tyack, 2001). Of great concern is the increase in the number of students who display severe problem behavior (Surgeon General's Report, 2001).

To be effective in supporting all students, schools need to implement a continuum of positive behavior support, from less intensive to more intensive, based on the severity of the problem behavior presented (Walker et al., 1996). This continuum includes positive behavior support at three levels: (1) universal, school-wide positive behavior support strategies; (2) targeted interventions for students at risk; and (3) individualized interventions for students engaging in severe problem behavior. The continuum of positive behavior support is detailed in Figure 2.1.

The triangle represents all students in the school and is divided into three levels of intervention. The bottom part of the triangle represents the approximately 80% of students who will benefit from universal interventions (Colvin, Kameenui, & Sugai, 1993; Sugai & Horner, 1999; Taylor-Greene et al., 1997). Universal interventions are implemented with all students, in all settings. The most popular universal intervention involves adopting a school-wide approach to discipline. A school that implements school-wide positive behavior support (1) agrees on three to five positively stated rules or expectations, (2) instructs students on the expectations, (3) provides reinforcement for following expectations, (4) provides minor consequences for rule infractions, and (5) uses data on a regular basis to determine whether the school-wide behavior plan is working. We recommend that schools have an effective school-wide discipline plan in place prior to implementing the BEP.

Given an effective school-wide discipline plan, we recommend the addition of an intermediate-level intervention system to support students at risk for engaging in severe problem behavior. In the triangle, the middle portion represents the approximately 15% of

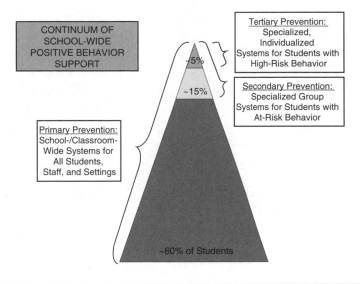

FIGURE 2.1. Three-tiered prevention model for school-wide positive behavior support.

students who will benefit from intermediate-level targeted interventions. These students may require extra practice in following school-wide expectations due to poor peer relations, low academic achievement, chaotic home environments, or a multitude of other reasons. Intermediate-level interventions are highly efficient "packaged" interventions that can be implemented with a group of students needing similar levels of support (Hawken & Horner, in press; March & Horner, 2002). The BEP, described in this book, is one example of a targeted intervention.

Some students will need more support than the BEP can provide. The top part of the triangle represents the approximately 5% of students who engage in the most severe forms of problem behavior and thus require intensive, individualized interventions. For these students, a functional behavioral assessment is conducted, and this information is used to develop an individualized behavior support plan (see Crone & Horner, 2003).

COMMITMENT TO PREVENTION OF PROBLEM BEHAVIOR

Schools across the country that have implemented effective school-wide discipline plans have experienced significant reductions in problem behavior and improvements in the overall climate of their school (Sugai & Horner, 2002). As a next step, schools should focus on students who are not responding to school-wide prevention efforts.

Consider the student who does not have a history of problem behavior. She begins acting out at school because her parents are going through a difficult divorce, and she could benefit from extra attention or support at school. In some schools, this student's behavior change might be overlooked because it is not severe enough to warrant a Student Study Team meeting or to involve the support of special education services. In a school with a

BEP system in place, a teacher, parent, or other school staff member could inform the BEP team that this student needs additional adult monitoring, feedback, and attention. Within 3–5 school days, the student could be receiving the support she needs. In a school without a BEP system, the student's behavior might have to become intense or chronic before she receives support. *By implementing a BEP system, schools are committed to preventing problem behavior. In essence, the school is reaching a student before he or she is in crisis and before the student develops a long history of engaging in problem behavior.*

COMMITMENT TO FUNCTION-BASED POSITIVE BEHAVIOR SUPPORT

In addition to implementing a continuum of positive behavior support, schools should be committed to designing interventions based on behavioral function (i.e., the reason why the student is engaging in a problem behavior). Students who engage in the same problem behavior over and over are usually either trying to avoid something negative (such as a difficult assignment or an unpleasant social situation) or trying to get something they desire (such as attention from peers or a teacher). Individualized behavior support systems that do not take into account the reason why the student is engaging in problem behavior may have little impact or may even make the problem behavior worse (Ingram, 2002).

IS THERE RESEARCH THAT SUPPORTS THE FEASIBILITY AND EFFECTIVENESS OF THE BEP?

Yes, research results support both the ability of schools to adopt and implement the BEP and its effectiveness in reducing problem behavior. A number of publications (Davies & McLaughlin, 1989; Dougherty & Dougherty, 1977; Leach & Byrne, 1986; Warberg, George, Brown, Chauran, & Taylor-Greene, 1995) support the basic approach of the BEP:

1. Define behavioral expectations.
2. Teach the expectations.
3. Build a regular cycle of checking in and checking out with adults.
4. Formalize consequences for problem behaviors across the school and home.
5. Collect information for ongoing evaluation and adaptation.

Three recent research outcomes, however, are of particular relevance.

Hawken and Horner (in press) report a systematic analysis of the BEP. Four students in a middle school were identified based on their ongoing levels of problem behavior and office discipline referrals. Using a multiple-baseline, across-subjects design, the authors examined the extent to which participating in the BEP was related to reduction of problem behavior. Results were gathered by direct observation in the classroom, and supported a link between use of BEP procedures and improved social behavior. The authors further documented that the school faculty and staff were able to implement the BEP procedures with excellent fidelity. Parents and students who participated in the study also reported that it was easy to participate in the BEP intervention. Overall, the data from this study demonstrate that the BEP can be implemented under the normal constraints in a school and that it is related to reduced levels of problem behavior.

These results have been examined in a more descriptive form in two additional studies (Hawken, 2003; March & Horner, 2002) in which many students in middle schools entered the BEP during a school year. The question of concern was *What percentage of students improved on the BEP?* The answer was that in both studies 60–75% of the students demonstrated decreased rates of office discipline referrals. There were students who did not improve, and, importantly, there were indications that some students demonstrated more problem behavior when they were receiving BEP support than when they were not.

In the Hawken (2003) study, the effectiveness of the BEP with 10 students was evaluated. Each student met the following criteria: He or she had not received BEP support for at least 6 consecutive weeks after the beginning of the school year, and then began the BEP program and received the intervention for at least 6 weeks following implementation. The results summarized the average number of office discipline referrals per week for each student before and after starting the BEP. For 7 of the 10 students, the rate of referrals decreased, and for 3 students the rate of referrals increased. For one student in particular, the BEP was associated with a dramatic increase in office discipline referrals and overall levels of problem behavior. It was clear that the BEP was not working for this student. This indicated two possibilities: This student was in need of more intensive, individualized interventions, or the BEP was contraindicated for this student due to the function of the student's behavior. For the other students whose behavior did not improve, only mild increases in referrals were noted. It may have been possible to conduct a brief assessment and modify the BEP to better meet the needs of these students. For a complete description of the study and results, see Hawken (2003).

A third study conducted by March and Horner (2002) examined, in more detail, how to avoid increases in problem behavior upon implementation of the BEP. March and Horner found (1) that students were less likely to be successful using the BEP if a functional behavioral assessment indicated that they did *not* find adult attention rewarding, and (2) that use of functional behavioral assessment information to adapt BEP procedures was successful in transforming intervention failures into intervention successes. Three students receiving BEP support were identified by March and Horner based on their continued levels of problem behavior after initiating BEP support. Each of these students received a formal Functional Behavioral Assessment (FBA), and the results of the FBA were used to adapt the instruction, rewards, or feedback procedures within the BEP. With these adaptations each student demonstrated both decreased levels of problem behavior and increased levels of academic engagement.

Collectively, these studies have demonstrated the following outcomes:

1. Typical schools are able to implement the BEP successfully.
2. Use of the BEP is functionally related to reduced levels of problem behavior, and, for some students, increased levels of academic engagement.

3. The BEP is likely to be effective with 60–75% of at-risk students.
4. Students who do not find adult attention rewarding appear least likely to respond successfully to the BEP.
5. If a student is not successful on the BEP, conducting a functional behavioral assessment and using the FBA information to adapt the BEP support can be effective in improving behavioral outcomes.

3

The Basic BEP

Critical Features and Processes

DEFINING FEATURES OF THE BEP

The BEP has several critical defining features that distinguish it from other targeted interventions and that increase its efficiency, effectiveness, and sustainability. These features include the following:

1. The BEP is an *efficient* system that is capable of providing behavioral support to a moderate-sized group of at-risk students (approximately 10–30 students) at the same time.
2. The BEP is continuously available within the school, so a student who is identified as needing support can get access to the BEP within 1–5 days.
3. The backbone of the BEP involves a daily "check-in" and "check-out" with a respected adult.
4. The BEP is designed to increase the likelihood that each class period begins with a positive interaction with the teacher or supervisor.
5. The BEP increases the frequency of contingent feedback from the teacher or supervisor.
6. The BEP requires low effort from teachers. That is, teachers should experience large changes in student behavior even though the individual teacher's BEP workload will be minimal.
7. The BEP links behavioral and academic support.
8. The BEP is implemented and supported by all administrators, teachers, and staff in the school building.
9. Students choose to participate and cooperate with the BEP system. They are not required to do so.

10. The BEP employs continuous monitoring of student behavior and active use of data for decision making.

Based on Behavioral Principles

The BEP is a school-based program for providing daily support to students at risk for developing serious or chronic behavior problems. The BEP is based on three "big ideas" from behavioral research:

1. At-risk students benefit from (a) clearly defined expectations, (b) frequent feedback, (c) consistency, and (d) positive reinforcement that is contingent on meeting goals.
2. Problem behavior and academic success are often linked.
3. Behavior support begins with the development of effective adult–student relationships.

Implementation of the BEP creates increased collaboration between school and home and increased opportunities for self-management. Each of these is also important for behavioral change by at-risk students. The administration and staff at your school will apply these three "big ideas" as they develop your BEP system.

A Brief Tour of BEP Elements

The elements and procedures for implementing the BEP are described in more depth later in this chapter. It is helpful, however, to have a general overview of the key elements.

1. *Personnel.* The BEP is managed by a BEP coordinator and a Behavior Support Team. All faculty in the school, however, also participate.
2. *Student identification.* A student is identified to enter the BEP by teacher nomination, family nomination, or request from the student. When a student is nominated for participation, an agreement is developed between the student, the family, and the BEP coordinator, and a BEP plan of support is defined. All students participating in the BEP choose to participate.
3. *Process.* The BEP involves a daily and weekly cycle. The daily cycle includes the following:

   • The student arrives at school and checks in with an adult (e.g., the BEP coordinator). At this check-in the student receives his or her Daily Progress Report (DPR).
   • The student carries the DPR throughout the day and hands it to the teacher or supervisor at the start of the day (for elementary school) or each class period (for middle school).

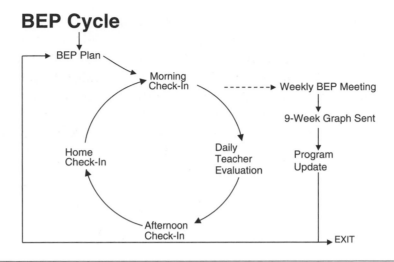

FIGURE 3.1. Illustration of the BEP cycle.

- The student retrieves the DPR after each class period or activity and receives feedback from the teacher or supervisor related to expected social behaviors.
- At the end of the day the student returns the DPR to the BEP coordinator, receives a reward, and carries a copy of the DPR home.
- Family members receive the DPR, deliver recognition for success and sign the form. The next morning the student returns the signed DPR to the BEP coordinator.

On a weekly basis, the Behavior Support Team holds a BEP meeting to review the percentage of points earned by each student and to adjust support options as needed. A diagram of the basic BEP cycle is provided in Figure 3.1.

Antecedent Features of the BEP

There are certain antecedent features of the BEP that increase its overall effectiveness. Antecedents are events or situations that occur before problem behavior, and can be thought of as the trigger that sets off the behavior. In order to prevent problem behavior, the key is to reduce the likelihood that it will occur at all by making adjustments to the behavioral triggers. The BEP creates a structure that eliminates antecedents to *problem behavior* by increasing antecedents for *positive* or *appropriate behavior*. These antecedent features include (1) provision of school supplies as needed at the beginning of the school day, (2) a prompt to have a good day, and (3) a prompt to have a good class period.

Disorganization is a common characteristic of the students on the BEP system. These students come to school without a pen or pencil, or without an adequate supply of paper. Coming unprepared for class is an antecedent, or trigger, for getting into trouble as soon as the teacher gives the class a direction. For the students on the BEP, this entire scenario can be avoided by checking to see if they have paper and a pen first thing in the morning and providing them with whatever materials they are missing before sending them to class. When a student checks in in the morning, the BEP coordinator reminds him or her to have a good day and prompts the student to remember the school rules. This daily prompt can mean the difference between starting the day out poorly or making better choices that start the day off in the right direction. Finally, students on the BEP also receive a prompt at the beginning of each class period (for middle school students) or at each class transition (for elementary students). This prompt reminds students of the class or school rules and helps the students keep their behavior on target during class time.

REFERRAL AND BEP PLACEMENT DECISION

Before a student can be placed on the BEP, at least two things must happen:

1. The student must be referred to the BEP. (Referrals typically come from a teacher, but they can also come from the student, a parent, or a member of the BEP team.)
2. The BEP team or the BEP coordinator must determine if the referral to the BEP is appropriate.

Referral Form

Each school should have a BEP referral form. An example of such a form is included in Appendix B. The referral form should include the student's name, the date, the name of the referring person, the reason for referral (i.e., description of problem behavior[s]), the hypothesized reason for the problem behavior (i.e., What does the student gain by misbehaving?), and the behavior strategies tried thus far. All the faculty and staff within a building should be familiar with how to use the form to make a BEP referral. The referral forms should be easily accessible and, once completed, should be given to the BEP coordinator. The coordinator should respond to the person who made the referral within 2 working days. If the student is to be placed on the BEP, he or she should begin it within a week of the receipt of the referral.

BEP Placement Decision

Not all students who are referred for the BEP will be appropriate for it. Some students will have mildly inappropriate behavior that can be corrected with slight modifications in routine. Some students will experience problem behavior in only one or two settings. For example, consider a student who repeatedly gets into trouble in the cafeteria line during lunch, but not during other times of the day. In this example, the student may benefit more from a change in the problematic setting than from a behavior monitoring system that tracks his behavior all day. The student could be dismissed to go to lunch 5 minutes early, eliminating the need to wait in line. Finally, some students may have behavior that is so chronic or severe that it cannot be remedied by a simple program like the BEP. These students will require more intensive, individualized behavior support (Crone & Horner, 2003).

Once a referral is received, the BEP team or the BEP coordinator will decide if a student should be placed on the BEP. In this manual we will discuss both a basic BEP process and ways to adapt the intervention. Adaptations and elaborations on the basic BEP are described in detail in Chapter 6. Typically, students are placed on the basic BEP program if they have attention-motivated problem behavior and/or if they find adult attention reinforcing. In some cases, the basic BEP may be ineffective or inadequate, and the BEP team may consider modifications to the BEP after a few weeks of implementation. Figure 3.2 presents a schematic for deciding if a student should participate in the BEP system and if the student requires modifications to the basic BEP.

The following section outlines the *basic* BEP process for an elementary and a middle school student.

BASIC BEP CYCLES

There are critical features of the process that must occur on a daily, weekly, and quarterly basis. The daily features involve both the daily participation of the identified students and the day-to-day management and implementation of the system. On a weekly basis the data should be summarized, reviewed, and used in making data-based decisions regarding individual students. On a quarterly basis, there should be a system for providing feedback to the teachers and staff, students, and parents on the impact of the BEP. Feedback should include a discussion of the impact for individual students as well as for the overall school climate. This next section details the critical features necessary at each point in this process.

DAILY FEATURES

Each student on the BEP starts and ends each day with a positive contact with an adult in the school and receives frequent monitoring and behavioral feedback throughout the day. In the morning, the students check in with the BEP coordinator. The BEP coordinator makes sure that each student has brought all of the necessary materials for the day (e.g., pencil, paper, and assignment notebook) and reminds the student to follow the school rules. The student picks up a BEP Daily Progress Report (DPR) from the BEP coordinator and begins the school day. In each class period, the student checks in with the teacher, who uses the DPR to rate the student's behavior within that class. In this manner, the student receives continual behavioral feedback and prompting. The DPR is turned in to the BEP coordinator at the end of the day. A copy of the DPR is sent home for the student's parents to review and sign—a simple strategy for including daily home–school collaboration.

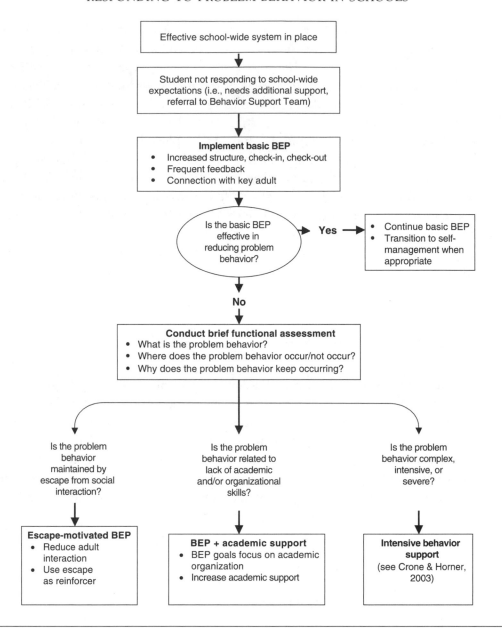

FIGURE 3.2. BEP schematic.

Middle School

Many schools will choose to create a BEP team to support the BEP. Due to personnel shortages, other schools may choose to rely on one individual to coordinate the entire BEP system. In our experience, schools that adopt a team model to support the BEP tend to be more successful at implementing and maintaining that BEP system than schools that have one person responsible for building and sustaining it. Similar to the process of working with students requiring special education services, a team approach is more effective in determining progress on the BEP, developing recommendations for modifications to the BEP, and planning for transition off the BEP system. Throughout this chapter, we will assume that a team model is adopted. We will make frequent reference to the BEP team. Schools using one person to run the BEP system should replace the term "BEP team" with "BEP coordinator."

It is easiest to explain the BEP process by describing the entire process for a sample student, whom we will call Jeremy. This was the first year of implementing the BEP system in Jeremy's middle school. However, the school had a backlog of discipline referral data. The BEP team examined the referral data from the previous year to identify students who might be at risk for problem behaviors in the new academic year. By using information from the previous year, the team could provide immediate behavioral support to at-risk students without waiting for a pattern of serious problem behavior to develop. The team identified several returning seventh-grade students who would probably benefit from the BEP.

Jeremy was a returning seventh-grade student who had received seven referrals the previous school year. Jeremy's referral summary is presented in Figure 3.3. According to his summary, Jeremy has a pattern of disruptive, aggressive behavior towards peers. His behavior occurs most frequently in crowded, less supervised locations, such as the gym, art and music classes, cafeteria, and hallways.

The BEP team decided that Jeremy would be a good candidate for the BEP. Two events had to take place before the team could begin to implement the BEP with Jeremy. First, the BEP coordinator had to obtain permission from Jeremy's parents. Second, the purpose and process of the BEP had to be explained to both Jeremy and his parents.

The BEP coordinator arranged a meeting with Jeremy's parents during the school day. Both parents agreed that the BEP would be a positive support for Jeremy. They were eager to have him start on it and were willing to cooperate and participate. While his parents were still there, Jeremy was excused from his classroom to attend the meeting. At this point, the BEP system was explained to Jeremy and his parents. The responsibilities of each party—Jeremy, his parents, and the school—relative to the BEP intervention were

Referral Summary Report

Student Name: Jeremy Walker

Behavior	Time	Date	Location	Referred by
Fighting	2:00	9/23/01	Gym	Gym teacher
Inappropriate language	12:15	10/17/01	Cafeteria	Lunch monitor
Disruption/noncompliance	1:15	11/2/01	Art room	Art teacher
Inappropriate language	12:00	12/08/01	Cafeteria	Lunch monitor
Disruption/noncompliance	10:15	1/17/02	Music room	Music teacher
Fighting	9:00	2/15/02	Hallway	Assistant principal

FIGURE 3.3. Summary of Jeremy's referral data.

discussed during the meeting. Also, a daily point goal for Jeremy was agreed upon by all parties. The goal for most students on the BEP is to receive 80% of the total points per day. For some students to be successful on the BEP, they may need to start out with a lower point goal (e.g., 60% of the total points), with the plan to raise the goal as the student experiences success. Everyone was given an opportunity to have any questions answered. Jeremy began the BEP the next day.

The school day begins at 8:30 in the morning. Students can do the BEP check-in between 8:00 and 8:30. At 8:00 A.M., the BEP coordinator opens the doors to the counseling office, and the BEP students begin to arrive. Because the students view the BEP as positive support, not punishment, many bring their friends to morning check-in. (Some friends even ask if they can be put on the BEP system!) The students who have been on the BEP system for a while are familiar with the routine. Morning check-in usually proceeds smoothly and efficiently because the routine is so predictable.

Jeremy arrives the first morning and is greeted by the educational assistant, who assists the BEP coordinator. She commends Jeremy for remembering where and when to show up. Every day, each student picks up a new DPR. Jeremy takes a DPR. The cards are printed on duplicate paper so that one copy can go home to his parents to sign, while the original copy is kept for school records. An example of Jeremy's DPR is presented in Figure 3.4. (A blank version of this form is included in Appendix C, and another example of a middle school DPR is shown in Appendix D.) Before leaving the check-in room, Jeremy puts his name and the date on the card. Next, the educational assistant checks to make sure that he has all of the materials he will need for the day. Jeremy opens his backpack to show her that he has loose-leaf paper, a pencil, a pen, and his assignment notebook. If students arrive in the morning without all of their necessary materials, the educational assistant provides them with a few sheets of paper or pencils and pens, as needed. Students are reminded and encouraged to come to school prepared the next day. After Jeremy has completed check-in, he is sent off with a prompt to have a good day and to follow the rules listed on his DPR.

Often, the students are given "High-5" tickets for checking in responsibly and being prepared with their materials. High 5's are part of a token economy system set up by the school to encourage school-wide support of the five school rules. All students have the opportunity to earn High 5's throughout the day for demonstrating appropriate behavior. A sample High-5 ticket is illustrated in Figure 3.5. (A blank version can be found in Appendix E.)

Once Jeremy leaves check-in, he has a few minutes before school starts. At the beginning of each class period, Jeremy places his DPR on his teacher's desk. All of the teachers in the school have participated in an in-service on the BEP, so each teacher knows how to respond to Jeremy's DPR. When a student brings a DPR to a teacher, it serves as an opportunity for the teacher to offer a brief positive comment or prepare the student for the class. At the end of the class period, the teacher rates Jeremy on a scale of 0–2 for how well he did for each behavioral expectation. A "2" means "Yes"; the student met the behavioral goal. A "1" means the student did "So-so," and a "0" means "No," the student did not meet that goal for that class period. Jeremy gives his DPR to each teacher throughout the day.

Daily Progress Report—Middle School, Example 1

(A- Day)   B-Day

Name: _Jeremy Walker_   Date: _9/18/02_

Teachers: Please indicate Yes (2), So-So (1), or No (0) regarding the student's achievement for the following goals:

Goals	1/5			2/6			3/7			HR			4/8		
Be respectful	2	1	0	2	1	0	2	1	0	2	1	0	2	1	0
Be responsible	2	1	0	2	1	0	2	1	0	2	1	0	2	1	0
Keep Hands and Feet to Self	2	1	0	2	1	0	2	1	0	2	1	0	2	1	0
Follow Directions	2	1	0	2	1	0	2	1	0	2	1	0	2	1	0
Be There – Be Ready	2	1	0	2	1	0	2	1	0	2	1	0	2	1	0
TOTAL POINTS	8			8			7			10			8		
TEACHER INITIALS	A.K.			B.D.			R.S.			J.T.			B.L.		

BEP Daily Goal   40/50   BEP Daily Score   41/50

In training _____   BEP Member _____X_____

Jeremy Walker
Student signature

Teacher comments: Please state briefly any specific behaviors or achievements that demonstrate the student's progress. (If additional space is required, please attach a note and indicate so below.)

Period 1/5 ____ _Behavior is improving!_ _____

Period 2/6 _____

Period 3/7 _____

Home Room __ _Excellent behavior today!_ _____

Period 4/8 _____

Parent/Caregiver Signature: _____ _Angel Walker_ _____

Parent/Caregiver Comments: _Keep up the good work!_ _____

FIGURE 3.4. Jeremy's completed DPR.

```
┌─────────────────────────────────────────────┐
│                 HIGH-5 TICKET                 │
│                                               │
│   Student Name: _Jeremy_____  │
│                                               │
│   Issued by: _Teacher_____  │
│                                               │
│   Date: _9/17/02_____  │
│                                               │
│                KEEP THE POWER!                │
│                                               │
└─────────────────────────────────────────────┘
```

FIGURE 3.5. High-5 ticket.

Teachers are encouraged to explain their choice of ratings to the students and to praise them on days when they meet or come close to meeting their behavioral goals (receive 2's on a majority of the goals). Teachers are also encouraged to hand out High-5 tickets to students who meet all of the behavioral goals in one class period. In this way, the BEP student receives continual feedback and prompting on his or her behavior. In addition, doing poorly in one class does not ruin the rest of the day. Each class period is a clean slate—a new chance to meet behavioral goals.

At the end of the day, Jeremy returns his DPR to the BEP coordinator. Both check-in and check-out are in the same location, so the routine is predictable. The BEP coordinator keeps the top copy and sends the second copy home with Jeremy for his parents. Checkout goes quickly, as many students have to get on the bus. However, it provides another opportunity for a positive adult contact. It also provides an opportunity to prompt Jeremy again for appropriate behavior. If students have met their goal for the day, they are allowed to select a small snack (candy, juice, crackers, etc.) to take with them.

Jeremy is expected to give the copy of his DPR to his parents. If he does not give it to them, they are expected to ask for it. There is a place for the parents to make positive comments on the card, sign it, and send it back. Jeremy returns the copy of the DPR to the BEP coordinator the next morning at check-in. This is a very simple way to increase the communication and collaboration between home and school—something that is always critical, but especially so during the middle school years.

Part of the BEP coordinator's job is to enter the daily BEP data into a database. It is critical that the school reserve enough time each week for the BEP coordinator to accomplish this task. The BEP coordinator collects the daily BEP data and enters the percentage of total points earned into a database for all of the students. This needs to be done on a daily basis or it is easy to fall behind. The daily data can be graphed to show each individual student's progress on the BEP. Students are held to a goal criterion of 80% of their points (goals may need to be modified, initially, for some students). For example, if 10 points were possible throughout the day, students have met their goal if they have received 8 or more points. Students who fall below this criterion have not met their goal. If a student goes for several days without meeting his or her goal, or if the student's performance is highly variable, the BEP team should see this as a red flag and should investigate, possibly modifying the intervention or increasing support for a particular student.

Figure 3.6 illustrates Jeremy's BEP data for the first week. It appeared that he struggled in the beginning of the week, but by Thursday he had begun to meet his goal of 80% of points. From this, the BEP team might conclude that Jeremy is beginning to adjust to the BEP system and that he has the potential to benefit from it. The team will continue to monitor and examine his daily data for patterns of behavioral success or struggle.

Elementary School

For students in elementary school, the BEP intervention is quite similar, but the DPR differs. The DPR reflects natural transitions of elementary school classrooms (such as the transition between reading and math) versus changes in class periods for middle and high school students. The behavioral goals need to be written in a manner that is understandable for younger students. The younger students may need visuals (e.g., smiley faces, thumbs up) to make it clear when goals are met and not met. Appendices F, G, and H display samples of DPRs for an elementary school.

Younger students may also need more practice to learn the routine of the BEP intervention. Students will not always remember to get their card in the morning or ask for feedback from teachers during transitions from one activity to the next. Teachers should provide support for students learning the program.

To demonstrate the differences between the BEP at the middle and elementary school levels, we will create a second example, that of Marisa Fernandez, a third-grade student. Marisa attends New Hope Elementary school. The school has had a BEP-type program in place for 3 years. This is the first year that Marisa has attended this school, because she transferred midyear from an elementary school on the other side of town.

Marisa's school records are late in arriving, so for the first 3 weeks of her attendance,

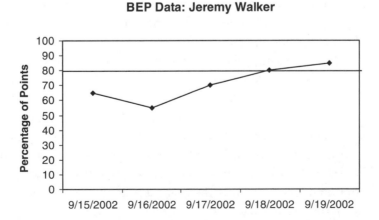

FIGURE 3.6. Jeremy's BEP data for the first week.

New Hope has no information about her academic or behavioral performance. However, by the fourth day of school Marisa is already experiencing frequent, repetitive behavioral difficulties. She has trouble finishing tasks. She gets into arguments with her female class-mates on the playground, and she frequently talks out while the teacher is presenting a les-son. Marisa's teacher, Mrs. Denken, makes a request for assistance from the BEP team.

After reviewing Mrs. Denken's request for assistance, the BEP team agrees that Marisa would be a good BEP candidate. Currently, there are only eight other students on the program, so there is plenty of room to add an additional student. In addition to reduc-ing her behavioral problems, the BEP intervention will help Marisa become better inte-grated into the school. She will meet more of the New Hope staff, and she will be taught the behavioral expectations at New Hope. She will have positive adult contacts on a daily basis. The BEP coordinator will make sure that she comes to class prepared with all the materials she needs for the day, including pencil, paper, and her daily planner.

Before Marisa could begin the BEP, the school counselor had to obtain permission from her parents. Additionally, the purpose and process of the BEP system had to be explained to Marisa and her parents. Both of Marisa's parents are Spanish-speaking, with limited English skills. New Hope Elementary has a high percentage of ELL (English Lan-guage Learner) students as well as staff who are bilingual in Spanish and English. Mr. Romero, the ELL teacher for the primary grades, was asked to attend the meeting between the school counselor, Marisa, and her parents. Mr. Romero was able to act as an interpreter and to clear up any concerns or questions that Marisa's parents had.

Initially, her parents were reluctant to have Marisa start the BEP. They were afraid that she was being identified as a "bad student." By working together, the school counselor and Mr. Romero were able to help them understand that the BEP would act as a positive support to Marisa rather than as a punishment. In the end, both parents agreed to have Marisa begin the program. After learning that there would be opportunities to earn prizes, Marisa was excited to begin. The BEP coordinator initiated the program for Marisa on the next school day.

Prior to beginning the program, Mrs. Saborski, the educational assistant who has been hired part-time to manage the BEP system, gives Marisa a "BEP tour." That is, the after-noon before Marisa begins, Mrs. Saborski walks her through each element of the program. She shows Marisa where to go for check-in the next morning, and where she will pick up her DPR card. She walks with Marisa to her classroom to practice giving a DPR to the teacher. They also practice giving a DPR to the lunchroom monitor and the playground monitor. By the end of the tour, Marisa feels comfortable with the new program.

At New Hope Elementary, the school day begins at 8:15 A.M. Students can do the BEP check-in between 7:55 and 8:15. Students are instructed to come to the library for check-in. At 7:55 A.M., Mrs. Saborski opens the doors to the library. Six of the nine BEP students check in with her between 7:55 and 8:15. The remaining three students are in kindergarten or first grade. Mrs. Saborski will go to their classrooms immediately after the 8:15 bell and check in with them individually. She found that it was difficult for the youngest children to remember to come to the library first, and that they would often be late to class when they came in for the check-in before class. The students in second through fifth grades appear to have no difficulty with checking in.

When Marisa arrives for check-in, she is shy and unsure. Mrs. Saborski asks one of the other BEP students to help Marisa. The other student reminds her where to pick up her new DPR card and then stands in line with her. Each of the students at New Hope has individualized goals, so each student has a separate folder with his or her name on it that contains multiple copies of that student's DPR card. The elementary school is able to have individualized goals for each student because there are so few students on the program. Individualized goals become more cumbersome when there are more than 10–15 students on the program. An example of a completed DPR for Marisa is included in Figure 3.7.

When it is Marisa's turn to check in, Mrs. Saborski praises her for remembering to come to the library. She shows Marisa the place where her behavioral goals are written and has Marisa read the goals to her. With Mrs. Saborski's help, Marisa writes the date at the top of her DPR. Mrs. Saborski asks Marisa to show her that she has paper, a pencil, and her planner. Marisa has her planner and paper, but no pencil. Mrs. Saborski gives her an extra pencil to use during the day. Marisa is encouraged to come to school prepared the next day. Like the other students, Marisa is given a "Chuckie-Buck" for checking in on time. (Chuckie the owl is the school's mascot.) Chuckie-Bucks are part of the recognition and reward program at New Hope. Students can put their name on the Chuckie-Bucks and put them in the raffle box at the entrance to the school. Every Friday the principal draws five names from the raffle box, and each of those students receives a special prize. After Marisa has completed her check-in, she is sent to class with a prompt to be on time and to meet her behavioral goals for the day. Often, each of the students is also sent off with a hug from Mrs. Saborski.

Once Marisa leaves, she has a few minutes before school starts. She goes directly to her third-grade classroom and is greeted by her teacher, Mr. Lee. Mr. Lee knows that Marisa is going to begin the BEP that day. He congratulates her on her good start and shows her how to put her card in the box for DPR cards on his desk. Mr. Lee waits for natural breaks in the flow of classroom activity to go over Marisa's DPR with her after each classroom transition. For example, after the students have completed morning activities, they begin their reading block. Marisa begins with silent reading. At this time, Mr. Lee talks with Marisa about the points she earned during morning activities. Some teachers find that it is too difficult to give students a rating after each classroom activity. Instead, they break the card down into two to four class periods (e.g., A.M. and P.M. or before morning recess, after morning recess, lunch/afternoon recess, after lunch/afternoon recess).

The rating scale for elementary school students can be different than for middle school students. In Marisa's case, the teacher circles a "happy face" if Marisa has met her goal and a "sad face" if she has not. All of the teachers at New Hope, including the specialist teachers (e.g., music, art) and recess monitors, have participated in an in-service on the BEP, so Marisa is able to bring her card with her to each activity she attends throughout the day.

As with the middle school, teachers are encouraged to explain their ratings to the students and to give them positive praise or Chuckie-Bucks when a student meets all of his or her goals for the class period or for the school day. If a student disputes a teacher rating, the teacher has been trained not to engage the student in a discussion regarding whether or not the rating should be changed. The teacher's rating is the final rating.

At the end of the day, Mrs. Saborski comes to each BEP student's classroom to pick up

Daily Progress Report—Elementary School, Example 3

Name: Marisa F.

Date: 1/11/03

☺ = 2 points
😐 = 1 point
☹ = 0 points

Points received _25_

Points possible _30_

Daily goal reached? (YES)   NO

Goal: 24/30 points

GOALS	Morning	PE/Music	Reading	Math	Afternoon
Keep my voice quiet while the teacher is talking.					
Say nice things or no things to other people.					
Follow adult directions the first time.					

FIGURE 3.7. Daily Progress Report for Marisa.

the DPR card and say good-bye. The students do not meet her in the library for check-out because there is concern that some students might miss their bus. Mrs. Saborski is able to get to each student because there are a limited number of students on the system and because the check-out portion of the BEP is very brief. Mrs. Saborski keeps the top copy of the DPR and makes sure that Marisa puts the second copy of her card in her backpack. Marisa's parents have been instructed to look for her DPR in her backpack when she arrives home. The check-out portion of the BEP is another chance for the students to have some positive time with a caring adult.

When Marisa gets home her parents pull out the DPR. Because the ratings are pictorial, there is not a language barrier in interpreting her performance for that day. Her parents are asked to sign the card and return it. They are also encouraged to write positive comments on it. Their comments can be written in Spanish, their first language. If there is any trouble with interpretation of the comments, Mr. Romero is able to assist.

After Mrs. Saborski finishes checking out with each student, she enters the BEP data into the BEP database. It is important to keep up with this on a daily basis. Some schools prefer to have each teacher be responsible for the entire BEP intervention for any students in his or her classroom. No matter who does the check-in and check-out, the key issue is that the data for each student should be examined frequently by either a behavioral team, a BEP coordinator, the school counselor, or someone who will be in charge of helping to make modifications to the program if the student is not making progress. Also, this team or person should be responsible for reporting progress to staff and parents about overall effectiveness of the program. Teachers want to know that their efforts are making a difference. There are many creative ways to make this work at an elementary school. It is up to the principal and the behavioral support staff to identify the strategy that works best for their school.

WEEKLY FEATURES

On a weekly basis, there are six primary goals to meet: (1) summarize weekly data for each BEP student; (2) prioritize students; (3) use data to determine if a student's BEP should be continued, modified, or ended; (4) award "reinforcers" to deserving students; (5) discuss potential new candidates for the BEP; and (6) assign tasks to relevant staff members. Each of these goals is discussed in detail.

Summarize Weekly Data

We believe the power of the BEP resides in two actions: first, providing continual, specific feedback and positive behavioral support to a student throughout the day, and, second, using data to make decisions. Once the data has been collected on a daily basis, it is critical to use these data for more than just a written record. It is easiest to use the data if one or two persons are responsible for entering the BEP data into a database on a daily basis. That is, at the end of each day or at the beginning of the next day, the BEP coordinator or a BEP team member enters the percentage of points earned by each student into a BEP database. For students who have smiley faces on their DPRs, numbers should be assigned to each face. For example, a student would receive a "2" for a smiley face, a "1" for a neutral face, and a "0" for a sad face. The database can be very simple. Most spreadsheet programs such as Quattro Pro and Microsoft Excel are excellent for organizing data and creating weekly graphs. An example of how to set up the database is included in Figure 3.8. The school can choose to use any software with which staff members are comfortable. As a critical feature, the software should have the capability to create line graphs from the database.

Once each student's data have been entered, it should be easy to create individual graphs to illustrate how well the student is doing on the BEP system. These graphs should be printed and brought to the BEP meeting, where the team can then review them. Figure 3.9 provides a sample of BEP summary graphs for six students.

Prioritize Students

Typically, the BEP team meets once a week for 30–45 minutes. In middle schools of 500 or more students, there may be as many as 30 students on the BEP system at one time. In-depth review of the data for each student within that limited time span will be impossible. A cursory review of all students is possible, but unlikely to produce useful results. Thus, the team should plan which students to discuss at the BEP meeting. We suggest prioritizing the students prior to beginning each BEP meeting.

After printing individual graphs for BEP students, the BEP coordinator can briefly review each graph. A visual inspection of each graph will quickly highlight which students are consistently meeting their behavioral goals, which students are consistently failing to meet their goals or to turn in their DPR cards, and which students are demonstrating variable performance. The BEP coordinator should choose about five students of concern to prioritize for the BEP meetings. Students who are not meeting their behavioral goals or who have recently demonstrated an abrupt, negative change in their BEP performance are good candidates. Each of the "priority students" is discussed in detail at the team meeting in order to make data-based decisions regarding his or her status on the BEP and his or her behavioral support needs.

	9/16/02	9/17/02	9/18/02	9/19/02	9/20/02
Student A	85	90	85	75	90
Student B		80			85
Student C	70	65	60	70	75
Student D	85	90	75	100	90
Student E	60	80	90	45	70
Student F	65	80	80	60	55

FIGURE 3.8. Example of a BEP database.

Make Data-Based Decisions

To read each graph, follow these guidelines. Each graph represents the data for one student. The graphs can be created so that they illustrate the student's data for only the preceding week, or for a longer period of time, such as the entire month or the entire academic year. Examples of long-term and short-term graphs are included in Figure 3.9.

Each graph represents a summary of the percentage of total points earned on the DPR each day. A data point at 80 indicates that the student earned 80% of the possible points. A data point at 0 indicates that the student earned 0% of the possible points for that day. Graphs should distinguish between 0% of points, failure to turn in a DPR, and school absences. In the sample graphs, an absence from school is indicated by the absence of a

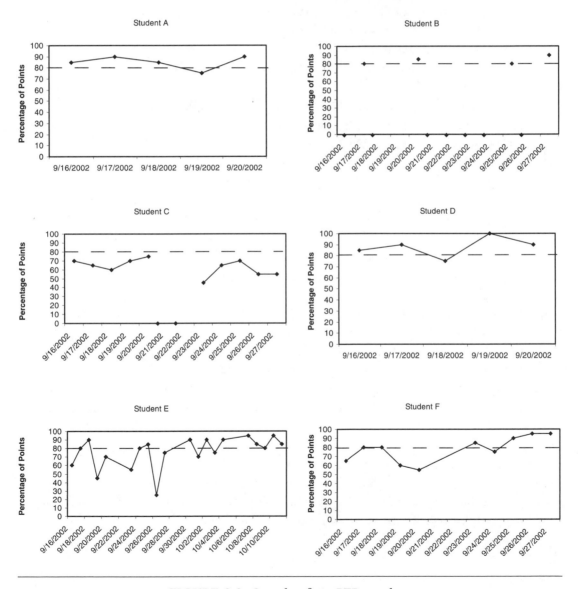

FIGURE 3.9. Sample of six BEP graphs.

data point for that day. Failure to turn in a DPR is indicated by an open dot at the zero mark. Zero percent of points earned is indicated by a closed dot at the zero mark.

The dashed line at the 80% point indicates the goal criterion level. Data points at or above the 80% line indicate that the student has met his or her goal for that day. Data points below the 80% line indicate that the goal was not met. The BEP team examines each graph to determine whether or not the student has consistently and actively participated in the BEP intervention, and is meeting his or her BEP goals.

Look at student A in Figure 3.9. This student is above the criterion level for 4 out of 5 days. It appears that this student has "bought in" to the BEP system. She is arriving every day to check-in and check-out and is meeting her goals in each daily class period.

Next, examine the data for student B. This graph represents the student's data over 2 weeks. While he also has met his goal of 80% of points on four different days, this is a picture of a student who has not bought in to the BEP system. He only has four data points for a 10-day period. The BEP team should question whether or not this student has completely checked out of the BEP system. That is, does he fail to pick up a DPR on most mornings, or does he decide whether or not to turn in the DPR based on how many points he has earned that day?

It is very easy to imagine that a savvy middle school student, upon seeing that he has only earned 30% of his points on a particular day, will choose not to turn in his DPR. Rather, he will tell the educational assistant and his parents that it "got lost" that day, or provide some other excuse. This behavior will be reinforced if there are no consequences for not turning in the DPR. The BEP team should be diligent about reminding students to turn in their DPRs and providing reinforcement for doing so, regardless of how the day went. One school we worked with implemented a raffle for students on the BEP. Raffle tickets could be earned for checking in and checking out on time. Students who met their goal at the end of the day received additional reinforcement, such as a snack to eat. Although not all students met their goals, they were motivated to receive a raffle ticket for a chance at the weekly drawing.

The graph for student C shows a student who is consistently participating in the check-in/check-out system, but who, day after day, does not meet his behavioral goals. The team needs to decide what to do with this student. *Has the BEP actually made his behavior worse? Do modifications or additional supports need to be added to the BEP?* The data help the team identify that the student is struggling on the BEP. The next step is to figure out what to do about it. In order to help them make this decision, the team may choose to look at additional data sources. For example, they may consider the student's discipline referral data or attendance record. Upon examination of all data sources, they may find that student C has received two discipline referrals in the past week for noncompliant behavior. This information, in combination with the BEP data, should set off a red flag: This student is continuing to have serious behavior problems. The BEP team should determine if additional supports or modifications could be made to assist him.

When presenting the student's BEP data, the BEP coordinator may choose to present the data weekly, as for student D, or cumulatively, as for student E. The advantage to presenting cumulative data is that it gives the team a broader picture of the student's behavioral progress. The disadvantage is that BEP team members may make mistakes when visually inspecting the data. That is, when examining student E's progress, they may conclude that he is not doing well because the picture is highly variable. However, if the team concentrates on the last five data points, they will note that the student has met his behavioral goal on each day and is actually doing quite well on the BEP.

Award Reinforcers

Sometimes the BEP team will decide to reward a student for improvement or for consistently meeting his or her behavioral goals. For example, student F has made considerable progress since he was first placed on the BEP. In the first week, his performance on the BEP was erratic. He met his goal only twice within 5 school days. However, in the second week, the graph clearly shows an improvement. In the second week, he is at or above his goal on 4 of the 5 days. Finding some way to reinforce this student for his sustained improvement will serve to maintain the appropriate behavior in the weeks to come. A simple way to provide reinforcers to students who have done well on the BEP is to provide a $1.00 coupon to the school store or snack bar. (A sample coupon is illustrated in Figure 3.10 and Appendix I.)

The power of this simple reinforcement system can be increased in two ways. The coupon can be signed and hand-delivered by the principal, who praises and encourages the student for his or her behavior. A copy of the student's BEP graph can be attached to the coupon. Providing the student with a graph of his or her behavior achieves several purposes:

1. It helps the student visualize and understand his or her own behavior.
2. It helps the student understand how his or her behavior is viewed by others.
3. It helps the student realize that someone is paying close attention to his or her behavior and that there is real meaning behind the DPR that he or she turns in each day.
4. It helps the student set goals and recognize whether he or she has achieved them or if he or she needs to continue to work on achieving them.

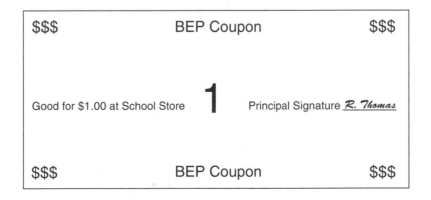

FIGURE 3.10. Sample BEP coupon.

Discuss New Candidates for the BEP

Another weekly responsibility of the BEP team is to discuss new referrals to the BEP system. In a school in which the BEP has been fully implemented, the teaching staff will be well aware of the BEP as a resource for managing problem behavior. The staff will need to have a way to access the team. This can usually be accomplished with a simple referral form. Refer to Appendix B for a sample. Once a student has been referred to the BEP, the team needs to decide whether or not that student should be added to the program.

This decision is guided by the following criteria:

1. The student is engaging in a repeated pattern of problem behavior in more than one setting or with more than one teacher/staff member.
2. The problem behavior has negative consequences on the student's social relationships with peers or adults, disrupts the student's education, or disrupts the education of the student's classmates.
3. The problem behavior is not dangerous to the student or to others.

Additionally, the team should consider how many students are already on the BEP. At the beginning of the school year, the team should assess their resources and determine the number of students that can be adequately managed on the BEP. Once they have determined a reasonable number of students who can be served by the BEP, the team should remain constant to that decision. We have seen schools that try to respond to every behavioral concern by placing the student on the BEP. As a result, the team and the BEP coordinator get overloaded, and the BEP system is not as effective as it can be when it is not run beyond capacity. It is critical that the team stay within the limits established at the beginning of the year.

If the BEP system is already filled to capacity but the team believes that a new referral will benefit greatly from it, they should consider whether other students are ready to be removed from the BEP. (A detailed description of strategies for fading students from the BEP is provided in Chapter 6). A frequent mistake is to keep students on the BEP indefinitely. One goal of the BEP is to help the student learn to gain control over his or her behavior, that is, to become a good self-manager. Maintaining the student on the BEP indefinitely promotes dependence rather than independence and self-management skills.

Assign Tasks

Each BEP meeting typically generates a list of "things to do." For example, if the team decides to add a student to the BEP, one of the team members will need to set up a meeting with the parents and the student in order to get permission for him or her to join the BEP and in order to explain what each person's responsibility is. Before the meeting ends, a team member should be assigned to this task with a deadline in place. If additional supports are decided on, someone needs to be in charge of implementing those supports. If the student is to receive a reinforcement coupon, someone needs to deliver the coupon to the student.

The team may find it helpful to use an Action Plan form to outline the tasks that need to be completed, by whom, and by what deadline. This Action Plan can be reviewed at the beginning of the next meeting to make sure that each task has been completed. Formalizing task responsibility in this way is one way to increase the likelihood that team members will remember and complete important responsibilities. The Action Plan form is illustrated and discussed in detail in Chapter 5.

QUARTERLY FEATURES

The critical features of the quarterly BEP process are twofold: providing feedback to the teachers and staff, and to the students and their families. It is important to provide feedback to these two groups for the following reasons: (1) to acknowledge the right of parents, staff, and students to be informed about their school or their child; (2) to maintain interest and involvement; (3) to recognize and encourage accomplishments; and (4) to point out needed areas of improvement (new goals) and achieve collaboration in meeting those goals.

Feedback to Teachers and Staff

Teachers and staff need to know how well the BEP system is running. *How many students have been served on it? Is there consistent participation from students? Is there consistent participation from teachers and staff? What has been the impact on individual student behavior? What has been the impact on overall school climate? What has been working well? What is still presenting obstacles? How can the teachers and staff contribute to improving the BEP system? Which students deserve recognition? Which teachers and staff members deserve recognition and appreciation?*

The team can be creative about how to provide this feedback to the staff and families. One school created a bulletin called "The BEP Gazette" that was distributed to staff on a quarterly basis. The bulletin listed the students on the BEP (identified by first name only) with a brief indication of their progress, provided reminders about meetings, and gave helpful hints on basic behavior management.

The bulletin can be distributed to teachers, staff, and families. It is important to preserve confidentiality, so individual students should not be mentioned by name unless they and their parents have given their express written consent. This is true even if the student is to be recognized for improvement. Remember, while it is exciting to be recognized for one's accomplishments, not all students may want to be publicly associated with a targeted intervention system.

Another way to provide feedback to teachers and staff is at staff meetings. The BEP coordinator or other representative of the BEP team can give a report on the BEP process and its impact. Students and families can be provided individual feedback at parent–teacher conferences. Both methods of providing feedback are convenient because both sets of meetings are already incorporated into the school's operating system. The BEP team takes advantage of existing meetings to achieve this important purpose.

TROUBLESHOOTING PROBLEMS
WITH IMPLEMENTATION OF THE BEP

What we have provided thus far is how the BEP works when it runs smoothly. Students check in on a regular basis, take the DPR to their teachers throughout the day, and check out in the afternoon. The student remembers to get his or her DPR signed by a parent. This scenario is not the case for all students. Part of implementing the BEP intervention involves modifying the intervention when it is not working for students or when the student is not participating in the program. Adaptations and elaborations to the BEP are discussed in Chapter 6.

4

Identification of Students
for the BEP

HOW DO YOU IDENTIFY STUDENTS WHO COULD BENEFIT
FROM A TARGETED INTERVENTION?

The best way to identify students for a targeted intervention such as the BEP is to have a system in place for regularly tracking discipline referrals. *Who has been referred to the office? How many times? For what problems? Under what circumstances?* If discipline referrals are systematically tracked and recorded so that it is easy to examine the data, meaningful referral patterns can be readily identified. The school may choose to "red flag" any student who has received a total of three or more referrals. (Depending on the average number of referrals per day, the school may choose a higher or lower standard for red flagging a student.) With a systematic, efficient tracking system, it would be simple to determine which students fall into the "red flag" category. A systematic tracking system also allows the school to easily determine which students are receiving the most referrals, under what circumstances, and for what types of problem behaviors. This information is critical to identifying those students who need behavioral support. In terms of evaluation, it allows for a comparison of the student's behavior before and after behavioral support was implemented.

Using Discipline Referral Data: Examples

Figure 4.1 illustrates the number of referrals received by each individual student. These data are taken from a school of approximately 350 students. There are about seven students who have been responsible for almost half of the referrals processed at that school. (Among them, the seven students have received 70 referrals out of 146 total referrals at the school.) These numbers are not unusual. On average, approximately 1–5% of the students in a school will have serious, chronic problem behaviors. These students will need intensive assessment and individualized behavior support. These are not the best candidates for a

33

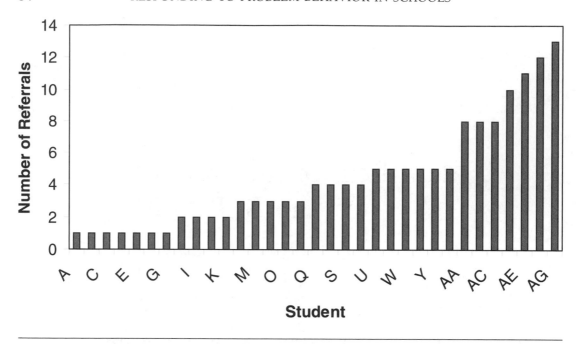

FIGURE 4.1. Referral data by individual students: 2001–2002.

targeted intervention. Rather, look at the 15 students who received three to five referrals in one academic year. These students may be at risk for developing more chronic patterns of problem behavior. It is likely that these students would benefit from a targeted group intervention such as the BEP program.

Figure 4.2 takes a close look at the referral pattern for an individual student. This student has five referrals. The figure summarizes the student's referral record. The student received three referrals for noncompliance, one referral for disruption, and one referral for inappropriate language. The student has a consistent pattern of engaging in mildly disruptive and defiant problem behavior. In addition, Figure 4.2 shows the times and places where the behavioral incident occurred and who issued the referral. This particular student has engaged in problem behavior across a range of settings with a range of staff. This student is a good candidate for the BEP. The BEP will provide behavioral feedback and support across each of the settings where the student has experienced trouble.

In contrast, the BEP intervention would be less appropriate for a student who received the same number of referrals if each referral originated in the same setting. In that case, it is more likely that the student's behavior can be improved by modifying the specific routine or setting associated with the discipline referrals. Once again, this is an example of trying to leverage your intervention so you get the biggest impact for the least amount of effort.

FOR WHOM IS THE BEP MOST APPROPRIATE?

The BEP is most appropriate for students who are considered "at risk" for developing serious or chronic behavior problems. These students consistently have trouble in "low-level"

Student Name: __Student W__

Behavior	Time	Date	Setting	Referred by:
Noncompliance	10:45	9/17/01	Social studies	Teacher
Disruption	12:15	11/20/01	Lunchroom	Lunchroom monitor
Inappropriate language	9:30	1/13/02	Hallway	Hallway monitor
Noncompliance	8:15	2/08/02	Math	Teacher
Noncompliance	11:00	3/12/02	Social studies	Teacher

FIGURE 4.2. Summary of referral data for an individual student.

problem areas. For example, they frequently talk out, come to school unprepared, talk back to the teacher, or cause minor disruptions in the classroom. In other words, their behavior is disruptive, detrimental to instruction, and interferes with their own learning, but is not dangerous or violent. The BEP involves a lot of positive interaction between students and teachers as well as increased monitoring of student behavior by adults at school and home. For this reason, the BEP will be most effective for students who engage in problem behavior in order to obtain adult attention or who find adult attention reinforcing. Students who are not reinforced by adult attention, or who even find it aversive, would not be good candidates for the BEP. For those students, the BEP could actually worsen their behavior.

The BEP is not adequate for students who engage in serious or violent behaviors or infractions, such as bringing a weapon to school or vandalizing the school. While those individuals might receive some benefit from the BEP, such students would require more individualized attention and support than can be provided by the BEP alone. These are the students for whom you are more likely to conduct a functional behavioral assessment (FBA) and to develop an individualized, function-based behavior support plan (Crone & Horner, 2003).

The BEP is not necessary for students who have been sent to the office on rare occasions or whose behavior is actually driven by a problem in the environmental setting. For example, school cafeterias can be loud, chaotic places. A student who is repeatedly referred to the office for yelling in the cafeteria is not an immediate candidate for additional behavior support. In a loud, chaotic cafeteria, the setting should be assessed and modified first. If the problem behavior continues, the student might then benefit from the BEP system or from individualized behavior support.

When deciding who is appropriate for the BEP system, it is important to remember that the problem behaviors of students eligible for the BEP will look different in elementary school than in middle school. A typical BEP student in elementary school might have difficulty taking his turn, refuse to share materials with others, have difficulty remaining seated or completing tasks, or be aggressive toward other students, especially on the playground or in areas with a lower ratio of adult to child supervision. A BEP student in middle school may be more likely to use inappropriate language, be frequently late to class, be defiant toward adults, or refuse to do work. *Whether in middle school or elementary school, the key is to identify those students who have a consistent pattern of problem behavior that has not yet reached serious or dangerous levels.*

HOW IS THE BEP SYSTEM INTEGRATED INTO THE SCHOOL'S OTHER IDENTIFICATION SYSTEMS?

Every school provides a range of services to students with diverse needs. For example, every school provides special education services. Many schools provide mentoring programs, extracurricular tutoring, or even mental health services. Each service typically involves a means to identify students who are eligible for, or need, the service. The more services available, the more cumbersome it may be to navigate the multiple identification processes. Adding a BEP system can further complicate matters.

School administrators should carefully coordinate the multiple services offered within a school. Each school should examine the identification processes used for each service and assess if any of the systems are inefficient, redundant, or overly bureaucratic. Representatives from each service area (e.g., BEP coordinator, special education teacher, and school nurse) should meet. They should determine how to reduce any inefficiency, redundancy, or red tape created by their multiple services. The key is to begin with awareness of what is provided by the other services. The next step is collaboration or partnership among the various services. Real collaboration among service providers in a school will reduce the likelihood that services provided by one group will be replicated, or even contraindicated, by another group.

Some schools find it helpful to list the existing committees at a school, along with the purpose of the committee and the staff involved. The "Working Smarter, Not Harder" graphic included in Appendix J can be used as an organizing structure for accomplishing this task. (Figure 4.3 illustrates an example of a completed Working Smarter, Not Harder organizer.)

Working Smarter, Not Harder

Committee, project, or initiative	Purpose	Outcome	Target group	Staff involved
BEP Team	Reduce problem behavior for at-risk students	Monitor daily behavior and reinforce appropriate behavior; build better relationships with school	Students with repetitive behavior problems	BEP coordinator, principal, representative sample of staff
School-wide climate committee	Improve school climate	Reduce behavior referrals, increase safety, increase organization and understanding of school routines	All students and staff	Principal, counselor, teachers, educational assistants
Discipline team	Provide negative consequences for inappropriate behavior	Individual students receive disciplinary action as necessary	Students with office discipline referrals	Vice-principal, counselor
School spirit committee	Increase school spirit and bonding to school	Organize pep assemblies, appreciation events, and other activities	All students	Interested teachers and staff
After-school tutoring programs	Provide opportunity for help with homework and other tutoring needs	Students receive small-group instruction in academic areas of need	Students with specific academic needs	School counselor and interested teachers and staff

Figure 4.3. Example of a completed Working Smarter, Not Harder organizer.

5

Getting a BEP System Started

Before implementing the BEP system, schools will want to be deliberate and well organized. They should be sure to lay a strong foundation on which to build a sustainable system and not rush haphazardly into implementation. It is much more desirable to wait until the timing is right and everything is in place so that the result is an effective system that will be maintained. Getting carried away with wanting to "implement change now" when the necessary groundwork has not been completed could produce the result that no one knows what to do, how to do it, why they are doing it, or what to expect from it. Once a system has been tried and has failed, it can be very challenging to convince teachers and staff to give it a second chance. It is critical to demonstrate effectiveness and efficiency from the beginning.

IS MY SCHOOL COMMITTED TO IMPLEMENTING THE BEP?

To implement an effective BEP system, it is important to assess whether your school is committed to this undertaking. Fill out the BEP Implementation Readiness Questionnaire (see Figure 5.1 and Appendix K) to assess whether your school has the critical features in place for successful implementation of the BEP. We suggest that the group of individuals who will become the BEP team fill out this questionnaire together. If the administrator is not expected to be a regular part of the BEP team, he or she should nevertheless be involved in this particular task.

The team should be able to answer "Yes" to each question before beginning to implement the BEP at your school. In addition, the team should be able to provide evidence that supports their responses. For example, if the team answers "Yes" to question 2 regarding staff buy in, then the team should be able to demonstrate concrete evidence of staff commitment. *Have they discussed the new system at a staff meeting? Were the staff polled regarding their interest and willingness to support the BEP? Did 80% or more of the staff*

Is your school ready to implement the BEP? Prior to implementation, it is recommended that the following features be in place. Please circle the answer that best describes your school at this time.

(Yes) No   1. Our school has a school-wide discipline system in place. In essence, we have decided on three to five rules, taught the rules to students, provide rewards to students for following the rules and provide mild consequences for rule infractions.

(Yes) No   2. We have secured staff "buy in" for implementation of the BEP. In essence, the staff agrees that this is an intervention needed in the school to support students at risk for more severe forms of problem behavior.

(Yes) No   3. There is administrative support for implementation of the BEP intervention. In essence, there is money allocated for the implementation of the program.

(Yes) No   4. There have been no major changes in the school system that would prevent successful implementation of the BEP intervention. Major changes include things such as teacher strikes, high teacher or administrative turnover, or major changes in funding.

(Yes) No   5. We have made implementation of the BEP one of our top three priorities for this school year.

FIGURE 5.1. BEP Implementation Readiness Questionnaire.

agree to support the system? Can staff members accurately articulate their responsibilities in helping to implement the BEP?

In our experience, schools that have implemented a school-wide approach to discipline are in a better position to implement the BEP intervention than schools without a universal system for behavior support. Without a school-wide discipline system, too much time is spent on managing individual student behavior problems.

In addition to staff buy in and commitment, administrative commitment is crucial as well. Administrators should be willing to participate in the development and operation of the BEP system. They should be able to dedicate the necessary personnel and resources to adequately support implementation. They should monitor the effectiveness of the program and encourage the BEP team to make improvements to the system as necessary.

Our experience in schools has taught us that implementing new interventions or attempting to change school systems when the school is undergoing too much change is likely to fail. When implemented consistently, the BEP is a powerful system to support students who are at risk for more severe forms of problem behavior (Hawken, 2003; Hawken & Horner, in press; March & Horner, 2002). If the system is implemented incorrectly or attempts are made to change a system that is unstable (e.g., teachers are threatening to strike, high turnover of administrative or teaching staff), implementation of the BEP system is more likely to be unsuccessful.

Commitment to too many projects at the same time is another threat to the successful implementation of the BEP system. For example, a school may choose to implement the

BEP, adopt a new reading curriculum, and initiate an on-site mental health clinic in the same year. With so many large projects beginning at once, the energy and effort necessary to build and sustain an effective BEP system may become too diluted to be effective. Thus, we recommend that implementation of the BEP be one of the school's top three priorities and that it only occur when the school is not initiating multiple new, major projects in the same year.

ESTABLISHING THE BEP SYSTEM

Once it has been established that your school is committed to implementing the BEP system, several things must be in place before the BEP system can operate on a daily basis. Each of these implementation features is listed in Table 5.1.

There should be personnel assigned to implement, manage, and maintain the system. Some schools choose to hire an educational assistant part-time to lead this project or assign the BEP to an educational assistant as part of his or her school duties. The key issue is that performing the BEP duties needs to be part of a person's job description, not an added responsibility without time allocated to do the job successfully.

The teachers and staff will need to decide what problems they will address with the BEP. They should identify behavioral goals that address those problems. Typically, schools choose to use their three to five school-wide rules (e.g., Be Respectful, Be Responsible, Be Safe) as the goals for the basic BEP. Students who have modified BEPs may have individualized goals.

Once goals are determined, school staff should decide on the system that will be used to track student progress toward those goals. More information will be presented later in this chapter on this topic. However, because one of the features most critical to the effec-

---

TABLE 5.1. Critical Features of the BEP

1. Personnel assigned (e.g., BEP coordinator) to oversee the implementation of the system.

2. Determine problems to be addressed by the BEP system:
   a. Academic
   b. Behavior (escape or attention maintained)
   c. Academic and behavior

3. Determine goals for students on the program.

4. System in place to track student progress on the BEP system.

5. In-service for all staff on how to implement BEP system.

6. Provide information to parents regarding program via newsletter, parent conferences, or orientation.

---

tiveness of the BEP system is using data regularly for decision making, it is important to know ahead of time how student data will be organized and summarized.

Prior to implementation of the BEP system, all of the teachers and staff will need to be adequately trained on the new behavioral support system. Most of the teachers and staff will have contact with the students on the BEP at one time or another. Each teacher or staff member must know how to appropriately participate in and support the BEP. This is critical. It is also critical to have the endorsement of the teachers and staff prior to implementation of this intervention. Without the participation, awareness, and support of the entire staff, the BEP system will not succeed. We also recommend that parents and caregivers be given information about the program. Some of the referrals for the BEP system may come directly from parents whose students are struggling academically or behaviorally and need additional support to be successful in school. Once these six preliminary features are in place, the BEP system can be implemented on a daily basis.

PERSONNEL NEEDS

In order to work effectively, the BEP system needs adequate personnel to run the program. We recommend that the school create a BEP team and a BEP coordinator. The primary responsibilities of the BEP coordinator are to (1) lead morning check-in; (2) lead afternoon check-out; (3) enter DPR data onto spreadsheets on a daily basis; (4) maintain records in centrally located, confidential location; (5) process BEP referrals; (6) create BEP graphs for BEP team meetings; (7) prioritize students for BEP team meetings; (8) gather supplemental information for BEP meetings; (9) lead BEP meetings; and (10) complete any tasks assigned at the BEP meetings.

BEP Coordinator

An educational assistant can carry out the responsibilities of the BEP coordinator. Most schools employ one or several full-time educational assistants, and the job responsibilities of an educational assistant tend to be more flexible than those of a teacher or administrator. Coordinating the BEP program should take about 9–12 hours each week. The tasks of the BEP coordinator and the necessary time allotted are illustrated in Table 5.2.

Leading Morning Check-In and Afternoon Check-Out

Morning check-in is the BEP students' first point of contact with the school for the day. On a daily basis, morning check-in provides the students with an ideal opportunity to start the day off well. Afternoon check-out is the students' last point of contact with the school. It is an opportunity to send students home with a positive attitude and a reason to look forward to the next school day. *The person who does check-in and check-out with the students must be someone that they enjoy and trust.* This person should be enthusiastic. When students look forward to seeing a person, they are much more likely to cooperate by checking in and

TABLE 5.2. BEP Coordinator's Time Allocation

Task	Frequency	Duration	Total time/week
Morning check-in	5 times per week	30 minutes	150 minutes
Afternoon check-out	5 times per week	10–15 minutes	50–75 minutes
Enter DPR data onto spreadsheet	5 times per week	20 minutes	100 minutes
Maintain records	5 times per week	15 minutes	75 minutes
Prioritize BEP students	1 time per week	20 minutes	20 minutes
Process BEP referrals	As needed	10–20 minutes	10–20 minutes
Create BEP graphs for team meetings	1 time per week	30 minutes	30 minutes
Gather supplemental information	As needed	30–90 minutes	30–90 minutes
Lead BEP meetings	1 time per week	30–45 minutes	30–45 minutes
Complete tasks from BEP meetings	As needed	60–120 minutes	60–120 minutes
		TOTAL TIME	9–12 hours

checking out on a regular basis than if they find the BEP coordinator to be dismissive, harsh, or punishing.

The logistics of leading check-in and check-out may seem complicated or overwhelming at first. All that is needed, however, is to establish a simple, accessible, predictable routine. Once the BEP coordinator has established the routine and each BEP student has been taught the routine, daily check-in and check-out will become almost automatic.

First and foremost, check-in and check-out need to occur in an established time and place. Imagine if the students had to remember to go to the counselor's office on Wednesday, the library on Thursday, and . . . look for a Post-it note on Friday to find out where to meet the BEP coordinator! These students are already struggling academically or behaviorally. There is no need to make the process more difficult by varying the location of check-in and check-out.

In terms of location, choose a setting that has enough space to accommodate the BEP coordinator and several students at a time. The setting should be centrally located but relatively isolated from other busy areas. For example, it would be difficult to conduct morning check-in in the main office at the same time that students and staff are trying to conduct the myriad interactions that occur first thing in the morning at most schools. Choice of location will depend on the resources available to the school. Some suggestions include the counseling office, cafeteria, or a family resource room.

Morning check-in should not last more than half an hour and should end before the first bell rings for school to begin. Students should not use participation in the BEP as an excuse for being late to their first class! Afternoon check-out should be even briefer, approximately 10–15 minutes. Many students will only have a few minutes between the dismissal bell and the time that their bus leaves the school building. The BEP coordinator might collaborate with the bus monitors to ensure that no students are left behind while doing BEP check-out.

Morning check-in consists of the following activities:

1. Greet each student individually.
2. Collect the signed (by parents) DPR from the previous day.
3. Check to see if student has loose-leaf paper, pens, pencils, and other necessary items for the day (provide extras to the student if necessary).
4. Student takes a new DPR, signs and dates it.
5. Prompt student to have a good day and meet his or her BEP goals.
6. Give student "High-5" ticket or equivalent for checking-in successfully.

The BEP coordinator may choose to keep a BEP attendance record or checklist of whether or not the student was completely prepared for morning check-in. A sample checklist is included in Appendix L.

Entering DPR Data onto Spreadsheet and Maintaining Records

The DPRs and the data gathered from them are helpful only to the extent that they are used. Completed and signed DPRs that are allowed to pile up day after day are only useful for filling up file drawer space. However, DPRs entered into a database on a daily basis can be used to monitor student progress, make data-based intervention decisions, and evaluate outcomes.

A simple database can be created in Excel or any other database software. (Refer to Figure 3.8 for an example.) Each student on the BEP is entered as a separate subject in the database with a corresponding line of data. Each day, the BEP coordinator adds the new date for a new column of data from the day before. The data are simple to enter. The percentage of points earned by the student is entered in the cell that matches the new date with the student's name. When data is entered on a daily basis, it should take less than 15–20 minutes to complete.

It is important to keep well-organized files. After the students' data have been entered, each DPR card should be filed separately into each student's file folder. Any other information relevant to the BEP (e.g., BEP graphs, permission slips from parents, or teacher interview) should be kept in the student's file as well. The files should be orderly so that it is easy to locate information. Maintaining the files should require 15 minutes or less per day.

Information regarding a student's behavior and treatment for that behavior is confidential information. While the student's files should be accessible for the BEP team members involved in working with the student, care should be taken to maintain the student's confidentiality. The files should be kept in a locked filing cabinet when not in use. A student's file should never be left lying out on a table or desk where other students or unrelated staff might have access to it.

Processing BEP Referrals for Assistance

Requests for assistance, or referrals to the BEP, will go through the BEP coordinator. The coordinator should have a stack of referral forms available to staff in an easy-to-access place. The referral should be simple and straightforward to complete. It then can be placed in the BEP coordinator's mailbox. He or she should briefly review the request. If any additional information is needed or if the referral is not completely filled out, the BEP coordinator should contact the referring staff member for more information. The coordinator will bring any referrals to the BEP team meeting. Using the criteria discussed in Chapter 4, the BEP team will decide if the student is an appropriate candidate for the BEP. Once a decision has been made, the BEP coordinator should follow up with the referring staff member to inform him or her of the team's decision.

Creating BEP Graphs for BEP Team Meetings

Prior to the BEP team meeting, the coordinator should create a BEP graph for each student on the program. Most database software can easily create line graphs like the ones illustrated in Figure 3.9. Printing graphs on recycled paper will save a great deal of paper over the course of the year. Putting multiple graphs on a page will further increase the amount of paper saved.

The coordinator can choose to graph only the data from the previous week or to include the students' data from a longer period of time. Whichever method is chosen, the data should be presented in the same manner for each student. Illustrating short-term data for some students and long-term data for other students may create confusion and errors in data interpretation by the BEP team.

It is helpful if each BEP team member can view his or her own copy of the BEP graphs. The BEP coordinator should make enough copies of the graphs to distribute to each of the team members. The majority of BEP team meetings will revolve around the "priority students." The BEP coordinator may feel that it is more efficient to only distribute graphs of the "priority students" to the team members, rather than a packet of graphs for all of the BEP students. In this case, the coordinator may find it useful to keep a master copy of all the student graphs in case questions regarding nonpriority students arise.

Prioritizing Students and Gathering Supplemental Information for BEP Meeting

Prior to the BEP meeting, the BEP coordinator should review data graphs for each of the BEP students. Many of the students will be doing well on the program, consistently meeting their goals from day to day. Other students may be performing poorly or may experience a sudden decline in performance. Some of the same students may be receiving detention or suspensions, or have poor attendance. The BEP coordinator will have access to this information as well. It is important to understand what is happening with these students and to determine if the students need additional supports.

The BEP coordinator should prioritize three to five students for discussion at the BEP team meeting. In addition to providing BEP graphs for each priority student, the coordinator can generate a copy of the student's detention/referral record, attendance record, or progress reports. This supplemental information can aid the BEP team in making data-based intervention decisions. The BEP coordinator may also choose to prioritize a student in order to follow-up on a previous decision or discussion.

Leading BEP Meetings

The BEP coordinator will lead the BEP team meetings. Each meeting will follow a similar agenda, but it is the responsibility of the coordinator to assure that each agenda item is discussed and resolved within an efficient timeline. The BEP coordinator brings the critical information to the meeting so that the team can discuss each student and decide on a plan of action. The team shares in the tasks or responsibilities generated at the team meetings.

Completing Any Tasks Assigned at the BEP Meetings

Multiple tasks may be generated from the team meeting. If a new student is added to the BEP, one of the team members will need to contact the parents for permission and an orientation meeting. If a priority student is not succeeding on the BEP, the team may decide to provide additional behavioral supports to him or her. For example, the team may propose a schedule change, curriculum assessment, or instruction on a behavioral skill. Once a plan of action has been decided on, someone needs to implement the plan. The BEP team members will share responsibility for coordinating the implementation of additional behavioral supports. Some (but not all!) of the responsibility for these tasks will fall to the BEP coordinator.

BEP Team

The primary responsibilities of the BEP team members are to (1) attend weekly BEP meetings, (2) contribute to decisions regarding individual BEP students, (3) conduct orientation meetings with students and families, (4) gather supplemental information on individual students, (5) contribute to student/staff development workshops and feedback sessions on the BEP, and (6) complete any tasks assigned at the BEP meeting.

The duties of the BEP team can be included in those of the team that currently exists to support students with problem behavior in the school. Some schools have Behavior Support Teams, Teacher Assistance Teams, or Student Study Teams that are currently addressing these students' needs. The goal is to not create additional meetings for school personnel, as time in schools is scarce. If the school already has a team that deals with behavioral issues, and if that team can devote 20–30 minutes weekly to the BEP, then that team can become the BEP team. If there is not such a team in your school, a new BEP team can be created.

The BEP team should incorporate a certain critical mix of individuals, including an administrator and a representative sample of the school's personnel. It is also helpful to have several individuals on the team who are knowledgeable about behavioral issues and who have had experience working with students at risk for severe problem behavior. Some schools choose to include each of their special education teachers on the BEP team. The actual size of the team will vary from school to school. We suggest limiting the size of the group to a maximum of eight in order to facilitate the ease of decision making and planning.

Getting the BEP Team Started

The BEP team will need time at the beginning of the year to develop processes and procedures. The three major tasks that must be completed are

1. Develop the Daily Progress Report forms.
2. Develop a structure for the meetings.
3. Develop the Request for Assistance forms and make decisions about the referral to the BEP process.

We suggest that the administrator set aside a half-day in-service prior to the beginning of the school year for the BEP team to make these decisions and create the necessary forms and procedures.

Developing Daily Progress Report Forms

The BEP team will need to decide what the primary behavioral goals will be for students on the BEP. We suggest limiting this list to three to five goals. Younger students (kindergarten to second grade) may respond more successfully to even fewer goals.

Developing Structure for the Meetings

The team should decide how to best use their time at each BEP meeting. We suggest creating a standard agenda that can be used at each meeting (see Figure 5.2 and Appendix M for a sample agenda). At each meeting, the team should discuss the three to five "priority students," whose BEP graphs and supplemental information should be reviewed. For each student, the BEP team should make one of four decisions: (1) remove from BEP, (2) continue to monitor progress on BEP, (3) provide additional (minor) behavioral supports or modifications, or (4) conduct comprehensive function-based assessment and intervention.

Figure 5.3 (see also Appendix N) illustrates a decision Sheet to remind team members of the discussion/decision process to follow for each priority student. *This decision should be made based on the data presented in the student's individual graph as well as additional information (e.g., office referral data, absences, detentions, etc.) that has been provided by the BEP coordinator.* Is the student meeting his or her goal on a consistent basis? Has there been a recent, dramatic change in the student's performance? Has the student stopped coming to check-in or check-out? *The data graph should be used to translate the student's performance and dictate the action that should be taken for that student.*

One person at the meeting should be responsible for completing an Action Plan form (Figure 5.4 and Appendix O). This form notes all of the decisions made and tasks assigned during the BEP meeting. The note taker should distribute a copy of the Action Plan form immediately after the meeting.

BEP Team Meeting Agenda

Date: _____   Note taker: _____

Team Members Present: _____

List of Priority Students:

1. Discuss priority students.

2. Discuss new referrals.

3. Identify students to receive $1.00 school store coupon.

4. Other BEP issues or students.

FIGURE 5.2. Sample agenda form.

"Priority Student" Decision Sheet

1. Look at BEP graphs.

2. Look at office discipline referral reports.

3. What subjective information do you have about the student from this week that adds to our understanding of the student?

4. Make one of four decisions.
   - Student is ready to be removed from BEP.
   - Things are going fine; keep on current BEP.
   - Having some problems—think of simple additional supports. (Who is responsible? Timeline?)
   - Having larger problem—student needs a comprehensive, function-based assessment and intervention. (Who is responsible? Timeline?)

FIGURE 5.3. Sample decision sheet.

ACTION PLAN

Date: _____   Student: _____ (Initials only)

Action Plan item: _____

Discussion:

Task	Person Responsible	Date to be Completed	Comments

Action Plan item: _____

Discussion:

Task	Person Responsible	Date to be Completed	Comments

FIGURE 5.4. BEP team Action Plan form.

After priority students have been discussed, the BEP coordinator will introduce any new referrals to the BEP team. The team will decide whether or not to add the referred student to the BEP.

Once new referrals have been discussed, the team can turn their attention to deciding which students should receive recognition for consistently meeting their goals over the past week or for demonstrating a significant improvement on the BEP intervention. These students can be rewarded with a $1.00 coupon to the school store or a similar reward.

Finally, if any time remains, the BEP team members can discuss any other issues relevant to the BEP process or other BEP students.

Developing the Referral Process

A sample referral process and sample referral forms were discussed in Chapter 3. The BEP team should have time at the beginning of the school year to individualize this process for their school. The team may want to make changes to the sample form, leave it the way it is, or develop a new form altogether. Whatever decision is made, it is important that the critical features of the referral form remain. The team should make decisions regarding who will collect the referral forms and who will decide whether or not a child is appropriate for the BEP program. *Should this be a team decision or should the BEP coordinator determine what to do with each referral to the BEP?* It may be helpful for the BEP team to create a flow chart that illustrates the BEP referral process. This flow chart should be shared with the staff at a staff meeting. A copy of the flow chart should be posted above the area where the blank Request for Assistance forms are kept.

Alternative Models of BEP Leadership

Some schools have chosen to divide the responsibility of the BEP coordinator across two individuals. The check-in and check-out and data management components are completed by an educational assistant, while the remaining team leadership responsibilities are managed by a school counselor or administrator. At times, educational assistants are uncomfortable with the leadership responsibilities of the BEP coordinator. Other team members may view an educational assistant as having less authority to be in the leadership position. Thus, splitting the responsibility across two individuals may be advantageous.

As a general rule, we recommend that more than one person be trained to manage each of the BEP coordinator's tasks. Because most of this work occurs on a daily basis, you need someone who can serve as a competent substitute if the primary BEP coordinator is ill or otherwise unavailable to come to work. The "substitute" may be another educational assistant or a BEP team member.

Not every school will have a BEP team. In these schools, the BEP coordinator(s) serves the functions of the entire team. This alternative model is more appropriate for small schools or schools with a small number of students at risk for problem behaviors. A school that chooses to forgo the team model must recognize that the BEP coordinator will be spending more time managing and implementing the BEP system. Without a team, the coordinator will be completing all of the assessments and implementing or coordinating all of the additional supports. *Effective administration of this model requires that a significant portion of the coordinator's job description be allocated for the BEP.* In our experience, implementing the BEP intervention using the team-based model is generally more sustainable than having a BEP coordinator in charge of the entire program and decision making.

RESOURCES

Time

One of the scarcest resources in the school is time. A second scarce resource is money. It is important to be well aware of this when planning to implement a BEP system. If there is to be a BEP coordinator, then adequate time and money must be set aside to make sure that the person can complete his or her job. This is crucial. Educators are some of the most giving people one can meet. Often, they will continue to give of themselves and their time until they cannot give any more. However well-meaning, a person who is stretched to his or her limit will lose the ability to be effective. If the BEP is to be a priority in the school, then some other program or job responsibility will have to be let go. The principal, in coordination with the BEP team, should make this decision.

Most schools expect their teachers and staff to participate on committees or in meetings. Participation on the BEP team can be counted for this required work. Team members should not have to do committee work above and beyond what is already expected of them. Time also needs to be set aside to teach students and staff about the BEP system.

Budget

The budget for initial and sustained implementation of the BEP will vary depending on the size of the school, number of students involved, and amount of employee hours needed for check-in/check-out, data entry, team meeting coordination, and other BEP coordinator tasks. Our goal is not to stipulate a specific dollar amount needed to implement the BEP, but to suggest the budget categories and offer at least one operating model budget. The key message is that resources need to be allocated to support implementation of the BEP.

Budget categories and the actual annual costs per category from one middle school with approximately 500 students is provided in Figure 5.5.

Staff and Student Commitment

A critical component of an effective system of behavior support is that the key people are aware of it and are willing to use it. If teachers do not know that this source of support exists, they will not make referrals, and consequently there will be very few students placed on the BEP. In addition, if teachers and staff have not been adequately trained on the BEP, they will not know how to respond when a student brings a DPR for their evaluation. It only takes a few inconsistent or negative responses from an adult for a student to lose interest in cooperating with the BEP. Lack of communication among the teachers and

Budget category	Category description	Example amount
Personnel	BEP coordinator (9–12 hours per week)	Per district pay scale
Materials	BEP forms on NCR paper	$250
	School supplies	$200
Incentives	Small rewards	$1000

FIGURE 5.5. Sample BEP budget.

staff in the building could put an end to the BEP system before it has a fair chance to work. Prior to initial implementation of the BEP, teachers and staff must agree to participate cooperatively in the system.

Equally important, students must understand what the BEP system is and how it works. This is true not only for the students on the BEP, but also for all the students in the school. When all the students in the school know about the BEP, they can support the BEP. They can support their friends who are on the BEP. The program becomes part of the school culture. When only a few students know about it, the program may be viewed with skepticism or ridicule. It may be viewed as one of those things they do for the "bad kids." Students tend to avoid systems that set them apart or give them a label.

The BEP must become a positive part of the school culture. How can this be accomplished?

1. *Begin by giving the BEP a high profile within the school.* Explain the BEP system to teachers and staff at the first staff development meeting of the year. Continue to provide this same in-service in subsequent years. Returning teachers and staff will benefit from the reminder. New teachers will be immediately integrated into the system. Also, explain the BEP system to the student body at the beginning of each school year.

2. *Always stress the positive aspects of the BEP system.* Talk about the BEP frequently in staff meetings. Give the teachers and staff quarterly updates on BEP student progress. Talk about the BEP at student pep assemblies.

3. *Next, ensure that the BEP is viewed as a positive support, not a punishment.* Publicly recognize students for their accomplishments on the BEP (with their permission). Use the BEP as a way for students to earn privileges. Publicly recognize teachers who contribute to the BEP. Publicly recognize and thank BEP team members for their hard work.

4. *Involve referring teachers and staff in the BEP process.* Teachers and staff members will "buy in" to the BEP to the extent that they experience direct or indirect benefits from the system. Increasing their contribution to the process enhances teachers' sense of benefit. After a referral is made, a BEP team member should contact the referring teacher or staff to gather pertinent information, which might include progress reports, work samples, a copy of the student's Individualized Education Plan (IEP), or a brief interview with the teacher. The point of contact increases the collaboration between the team and the teacher. It provides the team with a better understanding of the student, the problem, and the setting or routine.

The teacher and team members should communicate periodically about the student's progress. The team can provide the referring teacher with the data graph illustrating the student's performance and progress. The teacher can update the team regarding his or her continued concerns or satisfaction with the student's performance.

5. *Provide regular feedback.* It is important to provide regular feedback to the students, staff, and families. We all are more likely to believe in a program when we can see the real impact of the program. Regular, specific feedback to each group of key stakeholders in the BEP process is critical. Methods of providing effective feedback to students, staff, and families were discussed in Chapter 3.

TRAINING SESSIONS

Staff

Teachers and staff need to receive sufficient training in several elements of the BEP system: (1) making a referral to the BEP team, (2) providing supplementary information to the BEP team, (3) rating the student's behavior on the DPR card, (4) giving specific, effective feedback to the student, and (5) praising and encouraging the student for appropriate behavior. We suggest that training occur during a regularly scheduled staff or team meeting. Training can be delivered by the BEP coordinator or the BEP team. The teachers should be provided with copies of all the necessary forms. Opportunities to practice and to ask questions should be provided. Individual coaching should be made available to any staff member who needs additional training or support on how to use the BEP system.

Give booster sessions to remind everyone how the BEP works. Implementing a BEP intervention in a school is equivalent to asking the students and staff of the school to change some old habits. Whatever system the school has used in the past, they have had some method of responding to problem behavior. The BEP introduces a new strategy or a new habit. As with any old habit, initial change is neither immediate nor lasting. Both the staff and the students will benefit from "BEP booster sessions." A BEP booster session is an opportunity to remind all the key players of the purpose, process, and outcomes of the BEP. It is a good opportunity to answer questions about the program and provide feedback on its impact. BEP booster sessions can be easily incorporated into regularly scheduled staff development meetings or student pep assemblies. We recommend using booster sessions at least twice per academic year. The goals of the BEP and feedback on its effectiveness should be emphasized.

Participating Students and Parents

Students who participate in the BEP will need to be trained on how to participate appropriately. Their parents will also need to be given an orientation. As discussed in Chapter 3, we suggest that the BEP coordinator meet with the student and parents of each student who begins the BEP. This orientation meeting should occur *prior* to placing the student on the BEP. At the orientation, the BEP coordinator should explain (1) the purpose of the BEP, (2) the student's individual BEP goals, (3) how the DPR is used by the teachers, (4) how the DPR is scored, (5) how the school keeps track of the BEP data, (6) how the student will know if he or she is meeting the BEP goals, (7) what happens when the student meets his or her goals, (8) what happens when the student consistently misses his or her goals, (9) how to do check-in, (10) how to do check-out, (11) how to give the DPR to each teacher, each day, and (12) how to get a parent's signature and return the DPR each day. Students should be walked to the place where check-in and check-out occurs. They should be given an opportunity to practice and ask any questions they might have. On the first few days that a student is on the BEP, the BEP coordinator should take extra care to make sure that he or she understands the program and what is expected of him or her.

In addition to listening to the information provided to the student, the parents will require some information as well. The parents should receive a copy of the completed

DPR each day. They should be told to sign the DPR and make sure that their child returns it to school the next day. Parents should be encouraged to write positive or neutral comments on the DPR before returning it to school. It is important to emphasize to parents that the DPR should not become a means to punish the student if he or she does not meet the goal for the day. If punishment occurs, the student will soon start to avoid bringing the DPR home. Parents should be given an opportunity to practice and to ask any questions they might have.

6

The Modified BEP

Adaptations and Elaborations

The BEP is efficient because it uses a common organizing structure to respond to a group of students. Applying the same intervention for 30 students is far cheaper and swifter than creating 30 individualized responses. The efficacy of a common approach does, however, have limitations. The BEP may be an inadequate response to the behavioral needs of some students for a variety of reasons:

1. The BEP is contraindicated given the function of the student's problem behavior.
2. The BEP provides only one piece of the full spectrum of support required by the student.
3. The student is not an appropriate candidate for the BEP.

In this chapter we discuss BEP modifications and elaborations that address the first two issues. Identification of appropriate candidates for the BEP was discussed in Chapter 4.

WHEN IS A MODIFIED BEP APPROPRIATE?

The BEP team briefly screens all BEP referrals to decide whether a student is an appropriate candidate for the program. Once a student passes this simple screen, the student begins the basic BEP. Daily behavioral data is immediately available for each student on the BEP. The BEP team should consider a modified BEP if the basic BEP is ineffective. We suggest that the team collect BEP data for at least 2–3 weeks before considering a modified BEP.

Is the BEP effective for this student? The BEP team can answer this question if (1) the student has a specific, measurable, behavior goal, and (2) BEP data have been collected and recorded, consistently and accurately. Both criteria are easily met when the BEP system is implemented with fidelity.

For most BEP students, the measurable goal will be "Student will earn at least 80% of possible points each day." For students who are initially incapable of succeeding at this level, the BEP team may adjust this goal downward.

To determine if the BEP is working for a specific student, the BEP team examines the student's data graphs. *Is the student meeting his or her BEP goal on at least 4 out of 5 days? If the student is not meeting that goal, how discrepant is the student's performance?* The team is less likely to be concerned about a student who consistently earns 70% of points than a student who earns less than 50% of points on a daily basis. In addition to percentage of points earned, the team can look for other important patterns. *Does the student frequently forget to pick up the DPR in the morning or refuse to turn it in at the end of the day? Does the student consistently meet his or her goal on Tuesday, Wednesday, and Thursday, but have significant behavioral problems on Monday and Friday? What other data patterns does the team perceive?*

If the team determines that the program is ineffective for a specific student, they should brainstorm strategies for modifying the basic BEP in a manner that will improve its effectiveness for that student. For example, a student who is not picking up the DPR in the morning may have a difficult relationship with the person who runs morning check-in, and may be trying to avoid that person. The team may consider identifying an adult who has a special connection with the student. The student could check in with the other adult instead. A student who consistently refuses to return the DPR with a parent signature may be getting in serious trouble at home for less-than-perfect performance. The BEP coordinator may review the home component guidelines with the parent, or the team may decide to eliminate the parent signature requirement for this student. In this case, schools we have worked with have assigned the student to a "surrogate parent," such as a teacher, educational assistant, or janitor in the school. The surrogate parent will sign the form and provide the student with additional positive feedback on his or her behavior. A student who is earning 50% of his or her points on a daily basis is consistently utilizing the BEP, but the level of support provided is not adequate to meet the student's behavioral needs. The student may require additional supports, such as academic interventions or an individualized behavior support plan (BSP).

USING FUNCTIONAL BEHAVIORAL ASSESSMENT TO MODIFY THE BEP

One of the first steps in creating a modified BEP is to conduct a brief functional behavioral assessment (FBA). FBA is a method of gathering information about the events that predict and maintain problem behavior (Crone & Horner, 2003). This information can be used to determine the reason that a student acts in a certain way under certain conditions. FBA helps identify the *function* of the problem behavior.

Students' problem behavior can be broadly grouped into two categories: (1) problem behavior that is maintained by obtaining access to desirable stimuli (e.g., attention, activities, objects) and (2) problem behavior that is maintained by escaping or avoiding undesirable stimuli (e.g., activities, events, demands). FBAs can be fairly simple and brief, or complex and time-consuming. The complexity of the assessment will depend on the complexity and severity of the problem behavior. When used in conjunction with the BEP, we suggest conducting a simple FBA to identify the conditions most likely to result in problem behavior, and the consequences most likely to maintain the problem behavior for the identified student. A student whose behavior is complex or severe and who requires a full functional behavioral assessment (for the difference between full FBA and simple FBA, refer to Crone & Horner, 2003) will not be an appropriate candidate for the BEP. A simple FBA consists of interviewing one or more teachers. Typically, the referring teacher is the one interviewed.

Behavior Maintained by the Desire to Obtain Something

Students in this category engage in problem behavior because it results in obtaining something that they want. Students may want to obtain a toy, time to play on the playground, or attention from their peers or adults. The desire to obtain attention is a common function of misbehavior. Attention can be either positive or negative. For example, a teacher might reprimand the student in front of the class (negative attention) or a peer might laugh along with an inappropriate joke (positive attention). Some problem behaviors of these students might include talking back to the teacher, arguing or fighting with students, refusing to work, or disrupting the class.

Escape-Maintained Behavior

The problem behaviors exhibited by students in this category are often indistinguishable from problem behaviors that are maintained by the desire to obtain attention or other stimuli. The difference between the two groups is the function that the behavior serves for the student. Students in this group may be disruptive, talk back to the teacher, and argue with their peers in order to get out of a situation or to get away from a person. For example, a student who dislikes male teachers may throw frequent tantrums in male-led classes if she has discovered that tantrums in class get her sent to the office (and away from the male teacher). A student who has difficulty interacting with peers may be disruptive during lunch so that he is sent to the principal's office. By engaging in disruptive behavior, the student has been removed from (i.e., escaped) an unpleasant social situation. Students may also engage in disruptive behavior in order to escape a task that it too difficult, long, or boring for them.

Academic-Related Problem Behavior

Students with behavioral problems often have problems organizing and completing academic work. The problem behavior of students in this group is related directly to the responsibilities of completing academic tasks consistently, accurately, and on time. Students in this category have trouble with the following types of tasks: (1) bringing the necessary materials to class, (2) arriving at class on time, (3) completing assignments on time, (4) turning in assignments, (5) being neat and organized, and (6) following directions. For these students, problem behaviors arise because of poor attention, poor organization, or poor memory rather than defiance, aggression, or poor social skills. An FBA may demonstrate that the student would benefit from academic assessment and academic support in addition to the BEP.

MODIFYING THE BEP TO FIT THE NEEDS OF A WIDER VARIETY OF STUDENTS

The basic BEP works most effectively for students with attention-motivated problem behavior and/or for students who find adult attention reinforcing (Hawken & Horner, in press; March & Horner, 2002). The system is structured so that students receive a positive adult contact at least twice a day. Furthermore, students receive feedback on their behavior throughout the day. On a nightly basis, students receive parental attention to their school behavior. To the extent that teachers and parents attend to and encourage students' appropriate behavior, this behavior will improve. Slight modifications to the content or process of the basic BEP can improve its usefulness for students with academic-related problem behavior or escape-motivated problem behavior, as well as students with attention-motivated behavior.

Modifying the BEP for Attention-Motivated Behavior

The basic BEP may be inadequate for some students with attention-motivated behavior. Although the basic BEP addresses the appropriate function of the problem behavior, the intervention may not be strong enough to create change in the student's behavior. The team may need to elaborate on the basic BEP in order to help the student meet his or her behavioral goal. For example, the team may decide that this student needs more frequent feedback and attention than the basic BEP provides. The team may modify the BEP to allow for more frequent interactions between the student and instructors. Alternatively, the team may suggest adding a self-monitoring and self-reinforcement package to the BEP for a student. As a third possibility, the team may suggest adding more powerful reinforcers for the student. For example, the student may respond more favorably to attention from a particular individual. Perhaps the student has a special connection with the librarian or the school custodian. One modification that the team could build in is the opportunity to either receive feedback from this individual or to spend an extra 5 minutes with this person if the student meets his or her 80% goal for that day. Figure 6.1 provides an example of a completed contract for a modified BEP for a student with attention-motivated behavior (see Appendix P for a blank contract).

Modifying the BEP for Escape-Motivated Behavior

Responding effectively to this type of problem behavior within the BEP system requires creativity. If a student's problem behavior is motivated by the desire to escape authority figures, the student will not respond well to a system that significantly increases the num-

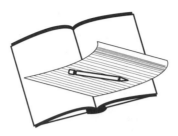

I, _____ Jasmine Jackson _____ , agree to work on these things this year.

1. _Be respectful toward teachers_

2. _Play safely on the playground_

3. _Keep my hands and feet to self_

I will work with Mrs. Jennings (music teacher) to keep track of my progress. I understand that I will have a chance to earn a reward each week when I meet my goals. A list of rewards I would like to earn include:

1. _10 minutes with Mrs. Jennings to learn to play guitar_

2. _Extra time in music class with Mrs. Jennings_

3. _Time to help Mrs. Jennings put musical instruments away_

I will try hard to do my best to meet these goals every day.

Jasmine Jackson
Signature of Student

I will do my best to help _____ Jasmine _____ meet his/her goals every day.

Mrs. Jennings
Signature of Coordinator

Mr. Jackson
Signature of Parent

FIGURE 6.1. Example of a completed contract for a modified BEP for a student with attention-motivated behavior.

ber of adult contacts throughout the day. In fact, this type of system could worsen the student's problem behavior (March & Horner, 2002). We suggest the following possible modifications:

1. Do not require the student to check-in/check-out directly with the BEP coordinator. Rather, the student can pick up a DPR from a designated box and return it to the box at the end of the day. The student is still responsible for giving the DPR to his or her teachers throughout the day.
2. The points earned on the DPR can be used to "purchase" personally meaningful reinforcers. For example, a student who has escape-motivated behavior might want to earn 5 minutes of extra gym time with a friend, as a way to escape a class that he dislikes. Another student may wish to earn reading time during a homeroom period she finds particularly boring. Prior to implementation of the BEP, a BEP team member can talk with the student to determine personally meaningful reinforcers and an exchange system for earning those reinforcers.
3. Even if a student generally avoids adult interaction, there may be one adult with whom he or she has a close connection. This individual may be utilized as the point of contact for check-in and check-out.
4. For some students, the function of the problem behavior may be to escape a task

---

Modified BEP

Attention Teachers:

Randall Prima will be placed on a modified BEP. The following modifications will be made.

1. Rate Randall's behavior on his DPR each class period. However, rather than discussing it with him, write your comments on the card and hand it back to him.
2. Randall will discuss his daily performance, and opportunities for improvement, with Mr. Reynolds, his football coach.
3. When Randall meets his goal for the week, he can choose from a range of personally meaningful reinforcers. Mr. Reynolds will coordinate the receipt of reinforcers.

Randall's reinforcers are listed below:

1. Time to work as office aide rather than attend homeroom.
2. Early dismissal from class one period per day.
3. 10 minutes' time in gym with a friend after classwork is completed, once per day.
4. Time to be peer mentor in younger-grade classrooms, once per day.

If you have any questions, please contact Chris Grayson, the BEP coordinator.

Thank you.

FIGURE 6.2. List of modifications for a BEP for a student with escape-motivated behavior.

that is academically difficult for them. In this case, the student may respond to the attention aspect of the BEP, but may require academic intervention as well.

Figure 6.2 provides an example of a list of modifications for a BEP for a student with escape-motivated behavior.

BEP Plus Academic Supports

A student who has significant difficulty with organization, task completion, and ability to focus may benefit from modified BEP *goals*. Goals listed on the basic BEP are typically behavioral in nature and broad in scope (e.g., Be respectful, Be safe). Goals listed on a modified BEP can be academic in nature, and more specific. The modified BEP could include the following type of goals:

1. Begin work immediately.
2. Complete assignment.

Daily Progress Report

Name: _____ Points Received: _____

Date: _____ Points Possible: _____

Daily goal reached? **YES   NO**

0 = No   1 = So-so   2 = Yes

Goal	A.M.	PE/Music	Reading	Math	P.M.
Begin work immediately.					
Complete assignment.					
Turn assignment in, on time.					
Arrive at class on time.					
Arrive at class with all necessary materials and books.					

Teacher Comments: _____

Parent Comments: _____

Parent Signature: _____

FIGURE 6.3. Example of a modified BEP with academic supports.

3. Turn assignment in, on time.
4. Arrive at class on time.
5. Arrive at class with all necessary materials and books.

In this case, the modified BEP acts as a constant reminder to the student about what he or she needs to do to succeed academically. This is helpful because many of these students have difficulty with memory or attention. Figure 6.3 provides an example of a modified BEP with academic goals.

The student may require academic support in addition to modified BEP goals. In this case, the BEP team may recommend that (1) the student undergo academic assessment to determine skill and performance deficits, and (2) the student receive academic interventions such as tutoring or after-school activities to remediate academic deficits. In a situation such as this, the BEP team recommends academic supports to the appropriate academic team. The BEP team is not responsible for providing the academic supports. For example, a student in special education may have an Individualized Education Plan (IEP) for a reading disability. The same student may demonstrate behavioral problems. The BEP and IEP teams will be more effective in producing behavioral and academic change for this student if they identify common goals, collaborate, and share relevant data.

FUNCTIONAL BEHAVIORAL ASSESSMENT (FBA)

The modified BEP will have the greatest positive impact when the modification is matched directly to the needs of the student. A mismatch between student and the modified BEP can, at the least, have no impact on the student's behavior, and, at the worst, cause the student's behavior to deteriorate. Due to strain on time and resources, most schools need to produce the greatest impact on student behavior in the most efficient manner. The appropriate BEP modification can be identified through effective assessment. *It is critical, however, that the assessment is brief and simple.* A complicated or time-consuming assessment procedure would eliminate the BEP's primary advantage, that is, efficiency of response. We suggest using FBA to identify appropriate BEP modifications for a particular student.

There are a wide variety of methods to conduct an FBA, ranging from a brief, semi-structured interview to a comprehensive interview coupled with observations in the classroom. To obtain the necessary information for the modified BEP, a brief or "simple" FBA is the most appropriate place to begin.

Simple FBA

The simple FBA is a brief, structured interview. The interview is conducted with the teacher(s) or staff member(s) who referred the student to the BEP team. The interview can be conducted by a BEP team member, school psychologist, behavior support specialist, or other person with adequate training and skill. The desired outcome of FBA is to (1) obtain an observable and measurable description of the problem behavior, (2) identify the setting events or antecedents that predict when the behavior will and will not occur, and (3) identify the consequences that maintain the problem behavior (O'Neill, Horner, Albin, Sprague, Storey, & Newton, 1997). This information can be used to determine if the student's problem behavior is escape-motivated, attention-motivated, or primarily academic.

There are several FBA interview instruments in print. Two similar instruments, the teacher interview of the Functional Behavioral Assessment–Behavior Support Plan Protocol (F-BSP Protocol) and the Functional Assessment Checklist for Teachers (FACTS) will be presented herein. Each school may choose to use a different FBA interview. An adequate interview includes the following critical features:

1. It can be completed in 20 minutes or less.
2. It identifies the specific problem behavior.
3. It identifies the routines that support problem behavior.
4. It identifies the "function" of the problem behavior. Each of the interview instruments discussed in this chapter meet all four criteria.

Case Example

The following case example demonstrates how to use the simple FBA to determine the type of BEP modifications that may be most appropriate for an individual student. In each example interview, the student and problem (i.e., incomplete assignments) remain the same, but the reason (function) for the problem behavior changes.

Background Information

Randall is a sixth-grade student at Fairview Middle School. He is well liked by the other students. He has a good sense of humor and is on several athletic teams, including soccer and baseball. Randall is struggling academically. On his most recent report card, he received a D in Math and failing grades in Social Studies and English. His poor grades in each of these classes are due primarily to a significant number of incomplete or missing class assignments. During the same grading period, Randall also received an A in Physical Education and a B in Industrial Arts. Randall is referred to the BEP team by his Social Studies/English teacher, Mrs. Nielsen.

BEP Plus Academic Supports

Mr. Jensen, the school counselor and a member of the BEP team, interviews Mrs. Nielsen. The results of the interview using the F-BSP Protocol are illustrated in Figure 6.4. In this interview the description of the problem behavior is the most revealing. As Mrs. Nielsen describes Randall's poor work completion, it becomes clear that he has trouble remembering to bring assignments and materials to class, is unorganized, and has trouble paying attention in class. He does not appear to be gaining anything specific from this behavior. For example, he sits quietly at his desk, not talking with or receiving attention from his

FUNCTIONAL BEHAVIORAL ASSESSMENT INTERVIEW—TEACHER/STAFF/PARENT

Student Name: Randall   **Age:** 13   **Grade:** 6   **Date:** 12/2/02

Person(s) interviewed: Mrs. Nielsen

Interviewer: Mr. Jensen

Student Profile: What is the student good at or what are some strengths that the student brings to school?

Has a good sense of humor, is athletic, and is well liked by other students.

Step 1A: Interview Teacher/Staff/Parent

Description of the Behavior

What does the problem behavior(s) look like?
Incomplete and missing assignments; Randall forgets to bring his materials (e.g., binder, pencil, paper) to class and often forgets his homework.
How often does the problem behavior(s) occur?
Assignments are missing on a weekly basis in Math, Social Studies, and English.
How long does the problem behavior(s) last when it does occur?
If Randall forgets his materials and homework it can disrupt the whole period because he is not ready to go over the homework and is unprepared for new lesson.
How disruptive or dangerous is the problem behavior(s)?
Behavior is not dangerous but is disruptive to his academic performance. At risk for being retained.

Description of the Antecedent

Identifying Routines: When, where, and with whom are problem behaviors most likely?

Schedule (Times)	Activity	Specific Problem Behavior	Likelihood of Problem Behavior	With Whom Does Problem Occur?
8:30–9:30	Math	Unorganized/Forgets homework	Low 1 2 3 4 (5) 6 High	Mrs. Singh
9:30–10:30	Physical Education		(1) 2 3 4 5 6	Mr. Woods
10:30–11:30	Social Studies	Unorganized/Forgets homework	1 2 3 4 5 (6)	Mrs. Nielsen
11:30–12:00	Lunch		(1) 2 3 4 5 6	
12:00–12:30	Homeroom		(1) 2 3 4 5 6	Mrs. Sanchez
12:30–1:30	English/Language Arts	Unorganized/Forgets homework	1 2 3 4 5 (6)	Mrs. Nielsen
1:30–2:30	Science	Unorganized/Forgets homework	1 2 3 (4) 5 6	Mrs. Avila
2:30–3:30	Industrial Arts		(1) 2 3 4 5 6	Mr. Carpenter

(continued)

FIGURE 6.4. Example of a completed F-BSP interview: BEP plus academic supports. The form itself is adapted with permission from March et al. (2000).

FIGURE 6.4. (*continued*)

Summarize Antecedent (and Setting Events)

> **What situations seem to set off the problem behavior?** (difficult tasks, transitions, structured activities, small-group settings, teacher's request, particular individuals, etc.)
> Classes that require homework and organization with materials.
>
> **When is the problem behavior most likely to occur?** (times of day and days of the week)
> During Social Studies, English, and Math. It also happens in Science but not as often due to the "hands on" nature of the class (not as much homework).
> **When is the problem behavior least likely to occur?** (times of day and days of the week)
> During P.E., Industrial Arts, lunch, and homeroom
>
> **Setting Events: Are there specific conditions, events, or activities that make the problem behavior worse?** (missed medication, history of academic failure, conflict at home, missed meals, lack of sleep, history of problems with peers, etc.)
> None identified

Description of the Consequence

> **What usually happens after the behavior occurs?** (what is the teacher's reaction, how do other students react, is the student sent to the office, does the student get out of doing work, does the student get in a power struggle, etc.)
> He receives reprimands from his teachers and parents, and ultimately receives poor grades. He's required to continue to do his work in class—does not get sent out of class.

- - - - - - End of Interview - - - - - -

Step 2A: Propose a Testable Explanation

Setting Event	Antecedent	Behavior	Consequence
	Classes requiring organization/homework (e.g., Math, Social Studies)	1. Doesn't complete homework 2. Comes to class without materials	Poor grades

Function of the Behavior

For each ABC sequence listed above, why do you think the behavior is occurring? (to get teacher attention, peer attention, desired object/activity, or escape undesirable activity, demand, particular people, etc.)

1. <u>When taking a class that requires homework, organization and materials, Randall appears to have difficulty remembering homework assignments and organizing materials, which results in poor grades in those classes.</u>

How confident are you that your testable explanation is accurate?

Very sure			So-so			Not at all
6	⑤	4		3	2	1

peers. He is not escaping work or the situation, as he is never sent out of the classroom and Mrs. Nielsen requires him to continue to work throughout the class period. In this example, it appears that Randall would benefit from a BEP with academic supports. The team could recommend at least three options:

1. Modify the goals of the BEP to reflect specific, organizational goals.
2. Conduct an academic assessment to determine the student's academic performance level.
3. Modify the student's curriculum and assignment to more closely reflect his or her skill level.

BEP Plus Modifications for Attention-Motivated Behavior

Now examine the interview presented in Figure 6.5. Mrs. Nielsen indicates that Randall becomes teary-eyed and withdrawn whenever he is given a written assignment in class. This behavior results in concern from his teacher and friends, who try to cheer him up. In the end, his assignments remain undone or incomplete. Information gathered from Randall's Math and Social Studies teachers confirms a similar pattern of behavior. Academic assessments indicate that Randall is capable of completing the assignments at the level they are currently provided.

This example illustrates the same student with the same concern, but it is clear that the problem behavior is not due to lack of organization and performance skills. Rather, the poor work completion serves a specific purpose for Randall. It provides a method for obtaining significant attention from both teachers and peers.

In this example, the basic BEP will address some of Randall's attention-motivated behavior. However, the basic BEP may not be sufficient because it does not address Randall's ability to obtain peer attention for inappropriate behavior (other students stop doing their work to look at him, help him, or console him). A modified BEP could include a way that Randall could earn peer attention for appropriate behavior. For example, the classroom could earn an award contingent on Randall's behavior. If Randall completes his assignment and does not cry or become withdrawn, the whole class could earn an extra 5 minutes of recess. In this scenario, students in the classroom would be expected to encourage Randall to meet his goal and to complete his assignment. Alternatively, Randall may feel too much pressure if the group's reward relies solely on his behavior. The teacher could remove some of this burden with a slight change. The teacher could say that the class will earn an extra recess if everyone in the class finishes their assignment on time. This requirement should have the same impact on Randall's behavior and the behavior of his peers, without putting undue pressure on him alone. Other ways to provide Randall with peer attention may include (1) providing a tangible reinforcer that could be shared with peers (e.g., tokens for the snack bar) upon meeting goals; (2) providing reinforcement to peers for helping Randall to be successful on the BEP; or (3) having him earn an outside-of-classroom activity contingent on successful progress on the BEP.

FUNCTIONAL BEHAVIORAL ASSESSMENT INTERVIEW—TEACHER/STAFF/PARENT

Student Name: Randall   **Age:** 13   **Grade:** 6   **Date:** 12/2/02
Person(s) interviewed: Mrs. Nielsen
Interviewer: Mr. Jensen

Student Profile: What is the student good at or what are some strengths that the student brings to school?

Has a good sense of humor, is athletic, and is well liked by other students.

Step 1A: Interview Teacher/Staff/Parent

Description of the Behavior

What does the problem behavior(s) look like?
Randall becomes teary-eyed and refuses to do work (sits with arms crossed, head down) when given a written assignment.
How often does the problem behavior(s) occur?
Four to five times a week when written assignments are given.
How long does the problem behavior(s) last when it does occur?
Randall cries and refuses to do work until friends and teachers console him (about 20 minutes); he then attempts the assignments.
How disruptive or dangerous is the problem behavior(s)?
Behavior is not dangerous but is disruptive to class and may have negative social consequences (e.g., other students have already started labeling Randall as a cry baby).

Description of the Antecedent
Identifying Routines: When, where, and with whom are problem behaviors most likely?

Schedule (Times)	Activity	Specific Problem Behavior	Likelihood of Problem Behavior	With Whom Does Problem Occur?
8:30–9:30	Math		Low ① 2 3 4 5 6 High	Mrs. Singh
9:30–10:30	Physical Education		① 2 3 4 5 6	Mr. Woods
10:30–11:30	Social Studies	Cries, refuses to do work	1 2 3 4 ⑤ 6	Mrs. Nielsen
11:30–12:00	Lunch		① 2 3 4 5 6	
12:00–12:30	Homeroom		① 2 3 4 5 6	Mr. Sanchez
12:30–1:30	English/Language Arts	Cries, refuses to do work	1 2 3 4 5 ⑥	Mrs. Nielsen
1:30–2:30	Science	Cries, refuses to do work	1 2 ③ 4 5 6	Mrs. Avila
2:30–3:30	Industrial Arts		① 2 3 4 5 6	Mr. Carpenter

(continued)

FIGURE 6.5. Example of a completed F-BSP interview: Attention-motivated behavior. The form itself is adapted with permission from March et al. (2000).

FIGURE 6.5. (*continued*)

Summarize Antecedent (and Setting Events)

> **What situations seem to set off the problem behavior?** (difficult tasks, transitions, structured activities, small-group settings, teacher's request, particular individuals, etc.)
> *Classes that require written work. Recent assessments indicate that Randall is capable of completing the work. He is organized, brings materials to class (binder, pencil, paper) and participates in class.*
>
> **When is the problem behavior most likely to occur?** (times of day and days of the week)
> *During Social Studies, English, and sometimes Science, approximately four to five times per week.*
>
> **When is the problem behavior least likely to occur?** (times of day and days of the week)
> *During P.E., Industrial Arts, lunch, Math, and homeroom*
>
> **Setting Events: Are there specific conditions, events, or activities that make the problem behavior worse?** (missed medication, history of academic failure, conflict at home, missed meals, lack of sleep, history of problems with peers, etc.)
> *None identified*

Description of the Consequence

> **What usually happens after the behavior occurs?** (what is the teacher's reaction, how do other students react, is the student sent to the office, does the student get out of doing work, does the student get in a power struggle, etc.)
> *When Randall cries, he is consoled by friends and the teachers, who say, "It's all right—you can do it," etc. A couple of times the counselor has come down to try to console Randall. Randall ends up not completing his work.*

- - - - - End of Interview - - - - - -

Step 2A: Propose a Testable Explanation

Setting Event	Antecedent	Behavior	Consequence
	Classes requiring written work (e.g., Social Studies, English)	Randall cries, crosses arms, puts head down, and refuses to do work	Consoling from friends, teachers, and sometimes counselor

Function of the Behavior

For each ABC sequence listed above, why do you think the behavior is occurring? (to get teacher attention, peer attention, desired object/activity, or escape undesirable activity, demand, particular people, etc.)

1. <u>When Randall is given a written assignment, he cries, crosses his arms, and puts his head down in order to gain attention from peers and teachers in the form of consoling (e.g., telling him it will be all right, etc.)</u>

How confident are you that your testable explanation is accurate?

Very sure			So-so			Not at all
6	⑤	4	3	2	1	

BEP Plus Modifications for Escape-Motivated Behavior

Finally, Figure 6.6 illustrates how poor work completion can be an indication of escape-motivated behavior. According to Mrs. Nielsen, Randall rarely turns in his homework assignments. When Mrs. Nielsen hands out an assignment, Randall will work very slowly, daydream a lot, and not complete his work by the end of the period. Mrs. Nielsen says that the work is not too difficult for Randall. He completes his work perfectly if the task is shortened or if he is told he can read his *Harry Potter* book once his work is completed. At times, when Mrs. Nielsen confronts him about his lack of work completion, he makes rude comments and stomps back to his desk. When Randall is asked to work on a worksheet in class, he announces that he thinks "This class is stupid." The other students rarely attend to Randall's outbursts. If Mrs. Nielsen presses him to complete the assignment in class, he may have a "blow-up" in which he throws his books on the floor, rips up the assignment, and yells, "I hate this stupid class." After a blow-up, Randall is usually sent to the office, where he is expected to sit calmly for the rest of the class period. A clear outcome of this behavior is that Randall is escaping an aversive situation—doing work in English class. It appears that his behavior is escape-motivated. Randall's Math teacher reports similar behavior patterns.

In this case, Randall should benefit from modifications to the BEP that address his escape-motivated behavior. Before a modified BEP can be effective, Randall's teachers and the administrative staff must make a commitment to changing their own reactions to Randall's behavior. His problem behavior can no longer be effective in allowing him to escape an academic task. Randall's teachers must commit to keeping him in class and expecting him to complete his work. If his behavior becomes so disruptive that he *must* be removed from the classroom, then the administrative staff must commit to having him complete his assignments while he is in the office. The inappropriate behavior must first be rendered ineffective. Once Randall no longer receives a reward (escape from work) for inappropriate behavior, a modified BEP can be introduced that allows him to earn personally meaningful rewards for meeting his BEP goals. Rewards should be determined through a discussion with Randall. Example rewards might include (1) leaving Social Studies class 15 minutes early, once a week, (2) working as a library helper once a week during Math class, or (3) being excused from one English assignment per week. Each of these strategies allows Randall to escape some work in Math, Social Studies, and English, in exchange for demonstrating appropriate, not inappropriate, behavior.

Figures 6.7–6.9 illustrate the same interview information in a different format. This structured interview is called the Functional Assessment Checklist for Teachers and Staff (FACTS). The FACTS is quite similar to the F-BSP Protocol interviews. The two instruments differ somewhat in format, but both are used to gather similar information. Either instrument is a time-efficient method to determine simple strategies to use to modify a student's BEP.

The BEP Support Plan illustrated in Figure 6.10 demonstrates how the information gathered in the simple FBA interview can be converted into specific strategies for the modified BEP.

Blank copies of the BEP Support Plan, F-BSP Protocol Teacher/Staff/Parent Interview, and the FACTS, along with instructions for completing the interviews, are included in Appendices Q, R, and S, respectively.

FUNCTIONAL BEHAVIORAL ASSESSMENT INTERVIEW—TEACHER/STAFF/PARENT

Student Name: Randall   **Age:** 13   **Grade:** 6   **Date:** 12/2/02
Person(s) interviewed: Mrs. Nielsen
Interviewer: Mr. Jensen

Student Profile: What is the student good at or what are some strengths that the student brings to school?

Has a good sense of humor, is athletic, and is well liked by other students.

Step 1A: Interview Teacher/Staff/Parent

Description of the Behavior

What does the problem behavior(s) look like?
Randall does not complete classwork (or homework) but instead sits at his desk, looks out the window, plays with objects. If pressed to do work, will yell, tear up things, and/or throw things.
How often does the problem behavior(s) occur?
Six to seven times a week, when homework is due or assignments are given in class that take an extensive amount of time to complete.
How long does the problem behavior(s) last when it does occur?
It can take all period to try to get Randall to do work.
How disruptive or dangerous is the problem behavior(s)?
Behavior is dangerous when he throws objects and is disruptive to the overall flow of classroom activity.

Description of the Antecedent
Identifying Routines: When, where, and with whom are problem behaviors most likely?

Schedule (Times)	Activity	Specific Problem Behavior	Likelihood of Problem Behavior	With Whom Does Problem Occur?
8:30–9:30	Math	Refuses to do work	Low High 1 2 3 4 (5) 6	Mrs. Singh
9:30–10:30	Physical Education		(1) 2 3 4 5 6	Mr. Woods
10:30–11:30	Social Studies	Refuses to do work	1 2 3 4 (5) 6	Mrs. Nielsen
11:30–12:00	Lunch		(1) 2 3 4 5 6	
12:00–12:30	Homeroom		(1) 2 3 4 5 6	Mr. Sanchez
12:30–1:30	English/Language Arts	Refuses to do work	1 2 3 4 5 (6)	Mrs. Nielsen
1:30–2:30	Science	Refuses to do work	1 2 (3) 4 5 6	Mrs. Avila
2:30–3:30	Industrial Arts		(1) 2 3 4 5 6	Mr. Carpenter

(continued)

FIGURE 6.6. Example of a completed F-BSP interview: Escape-motivated behavior. The form itself is adapted with permission from March et al. (2000).

FIGURE 6.6. (*continued*)

Summarize Antecedent (and Setting Events)

> **What situations seem to set off the problem behavior?** (difficult tasks, transitions, structured activities, small-group settings, teacher's request, particular individuals, etc.)
> *When asked to do work or turn in homework, particularly lengthy assignments*
>
> **When is the problem behavior most likely to occur?** (times of day and days of the week)
> *During Social Studies, Math, English, and sometimes Science*
>
> **When is the problem behavior least likely to occur?** (times of day and days of the week)
> *During P.E., Industrial Arts, lunch, and homeroom*
>
> **Setting Events: Are there specific conditions, events, or activities that make the problem behavior worse?** (missed medication, history of academic failure, conflict at home, missed meals, lack of sleep, history of problems with peers, etc.)
> *None identified*

Description of the Consequence

> **What usually happens after the behavior occurs?** (what is the teacher's reaction, how do other students react, is the student sent to the office, does the student get out of doing work, does the student get in a power struggle, etc.)
> *When Randall refuses to do work, he will sit, look out the window, etc., and when pressed to do work he will yell ("This is stupid!") and at times, throw books and tear up assignments. Sometimes he is sent to the office. He is able to get out of doing work when he engages in these behaviors.*

- - - - - - End of Interview - - - - - -

Step 2A: Propose a Testable Explanation

Setting Event	Antecedent	Behavior	Consequence
	Instructed to do work	Refuses to do work and yells/throws objects if pressed to do work	Does not complete work Ultimately sent to office

Function of the Behavior

For each ABC sequence listed above, why do you think the behavior is occurring? (to get teacher attention, peer attention, desired object/activity, or escape undesirable activity, demand, particular people, etc.)

1. *When Randall is given an assignment, he looks out the window, plays with objects, and ultimately ends up escaping the work that was required for the class.*

How confident are you that your testable explanation is accurate?

Very sure		So-so			Not at all
6	⑤	4	3	2	1

FACTS–Part A

Student/Grade: _Randall – 6th_   **Date:** _12/6/02_
Interviewer: _Mr. Jensen_   **Respondent(s):** _Mrs. Nielsen_

Student profile: Please identify at least three strengths or contributions the student brings to school.

Athletic, liked by peers, and good sense of humor

Problem Behavior(s): Identify problem behaviors

___ Tardy	___ Inappropriate language	___ Disruptive	___ Theft
___ Unresponsive	___ Fight/Physical aggression	___ Insubordination	___ Vandalism
___ Withdrawn	___ Verbal harassment	_X_ Work not done	___ Other _____
	___ Verbally inappropriate		

Describe problem behavior: _Randall forgets to bring his materials (e.g., binder, pencil, paper) to class and often forgets his homework._

Identifying Routines: Where, When, and With Whom Problem Behaviors Are Most Likely.

Schedule (Times)	Activity	With Whom Does Problem Occur?	Likelihood of Problem Behavior	Specific Problem Behavior
8:30–9:30	Math	Mrs. Singh	Low High 1 2 3 4 ⑤ 6	Unorganized/ Forgets homework
9:30–10:30	Physical Education	Mr. Woods	① 2 3 4 5 6	
10:30–11:30	Social Studies	Mrs. Nielsen	1 2 3 4 5 ⑥	Unorganized/ Forgets homework
11:30–12:00	Lunch		① 2 3 4 5 6	
12:00–12:30	Homeroom	Mr. Sanchez	① 2 3 4 5 6	
12:30–1:30	English/Language Arts	Mrs. Nielsen	1 2 3 4 5 ⑥	Unorganized/ Forgets homework
1:30–2:30	Science	Mrs. Avila	1 2 3 ④ 5 6	Unorganized/ Forgets homework
2:30–3:30	Industrial Arts	Mr. Carpenter	1 ② 3 4 5 6	
			1 2 3 4 5 6	

Select one to three routines for further assessment. Select routines based on (1) similarity of activities (conditions) with ratings of 4, 5, or 6 and (2) similarity of problem behavior(s). Complete the FACTS–Part B for each routine identified.

(continued)

FIGURE 6.7. Example of a complete FACTS interview: BEP plus academic supports. The form itself is adapted with permission from March et al. (2000).

FIGURE 6.7. (*continued*)

FACTS–Part B

Student/Grade: _Randall – 6th_   Date: _12/6/02_

Interviewer: _Mr. Jensen_   Respondent(s): _Mrs. Nielsen_

Routine/Activities/Context: Which routine (only one) from the FACTS–Part A is assessed?

Routine/Activities/Context	Problem Behavior
Classes that require homework and organization with materials.	Does not complete work.

Provide more detail about the problem behavior(s):

What does the problem behavior(s) look like?
Incomplete and missing assignments; Randall forgets to bring his materials (e.g., binder, pencil, paper) to class and often forgets his homework.

How often does the problem behavior(s) occur?
Assignments are missing on a weekly basis in Math, Social Studies, and English.

How long does the problem behavior(s) last when it does occur?
If Randall forgets his materials and homework it can disrupt the whole period because he is not ready to go over the homework and is unprepared for the new lesson.

What is the intensity/level of danger of the problem behavior(s)?
Behavior is not dangerous but is disruptive to his academic performance. At risk for being retained.

What are the events that predict when the problem behavior(s) will occur?

Related Issues (Setting Events)		Environmental Features	
___ illness	Other: _____	___ reprimand/correction	_X_ structured activity
___ drug use	_____	___ physical demands	___ unstructured time
___ negative social	_____	___ socially isolated	___ tasks too boring
___ conflict at home	_____	___ with peers	___ activity too long
___ academic failure	_____	___ other	___ tasks too difficult

What consequences are most likely to maintain the problem behavior(s)?

Things That Are Obtained		Things Avoided or Escaped From	
___ adult attention	Other: _Homework_	___ hard tasks	Other: _____
___ peer attention	_incomplete and_	___ reprimands	_____
___ preferred activity	_poor grades_	___ peer negatives	_____
___ money/things	_____	___ physical effort	_____

SUMMARY OF BEHAVIOR

Identify the summary that will be used to build a plan of behavior support

Setting Events and Predictors	Problem Behavior(s)	Maintaining Consequence(s)
Classes requiring organization/ homework (e.g., Math, Social Studies)	1. Lack of homework 2. Lack of materials	Poor grades

How confident are you that the Summary of Behavior is accurate?

Not very confident					Very confident
1	2	3	4	⑤	6

What current efforts have been used to control the problem behavior?

Strategies for Preventing Problem Behavior		Consequences for Problem Behavior	
___ schedule change	Other: _____	_X_ reprimand	Other: _____
_X_ seating change	_____	___ office referral	_____
___ curriculum change	_____	___ detention	_____

FACTS–Part A

Student/Grade: <u>Randall – 6th</u>   Date: <u>12/6/02</u>

Interviewer: <u>Mr. Jensen</u>   Respondent(s): <u>Mrs. Nielsen</u>

Student profile: Please identify at least three strengths or contributions the student brings to school.

<u>Athletic, liked by peers, and good sense of humor</u>

Problem Behavior(s): Identify problem behaviors

___ Tardy	___ Inappropriate language	___ Disruptive	___ Theft
___ Unresponsive	___ Fight/Physical aggression	___ Insubordination	___ Vandalism
_x_ Withdrawn	___ Verbal harassment	_x_ Work not done	___ Other_____
	___ Verbally inappropriate	___ Self-injury	

Describe problem behavior: <u>Randall becomes teary-eyed and refuses to do work (sits with arms crossed, head down) when given a writing assignment.</u>

Identifying Routines: Where, When, and With Whom Problem Behaviors Are Most Likely.

Schedule (Times)	Activity	With Whom Does Problem Occur?	Likelihood of Problem Behavior	Specific Problem Behavior
8:30–9:30	Math	Mrs. Singh	Low High ① 2 3 4 5 6	Cries, refuses to do work
9:30–10:30	Physical Education	Mr. Woods	① 2 3 4 5 6	
10:30–11:30	Social Studies	Mrs. Nielsen	1 2 3 4 ⑤ 6	Cries, refuses to do work
11:30–12:00	Lunch		① 2 3 4 5 6	
12:00–12:30	Homeroom	Mr. Sanchez	① 2 3 4 5 6	
12:30–1:30	English/Language Arts	Mrs. Nielsen	1 2 3 4 5 ⑥	Cries, refuses to do work
1:30–2:30	Science	Mrs. Avila	1 ② 3 4 5 6	Cries, refuses to do work
2:30–3:30	Industrial Arts	Mr. Carpenter	① 2 3 4 5 6	
			1 2 3 4 5 6	

Select one to three routines for further assessment. Select routines based on (1) similarity of activities (conditions) with ratings of 4, 5, or 6 and (2) similarity of problem behavior(s). Complete the FACTS–Part B for each routine identified.

(continued)

FIGURE 6.8. Example of a completed FACTS interview: Attention-motivated behavior. The form itself is adapted with permission from March et al. (2000).

FIGURE 6.8. (*continued*)

FACTS–Part B

Student/Grade: Randall – 6th   **Date:** 12/6/02

Interviewer: Mr. Jensen   **Respondent(s):** Mrs. Nielsen

Routine/Activities/Context: Which routine (only one) from the FACTS–Part A is assessed?

Routine/Activities/Context	Problem Behavior
Classes that require written work	Does not complete work and cries

Provide more detail about the problem behavior(s):

What does the problem behavior(s) look like?
Classes that require written work. Recent assessments indicate that Randall is capable of completing the work. He is organized, brings materials to class (binder, pencil, paper), and participates in class.

How often does the problem behavior(s) occur?
During Social Studies, English, and sometimes Science, approximately four to five times per week

How long does the problem behavior(s) last when it does occur?
Randall cries and refuses to do work until friends and teachers console him (about 20 minutes); he then attempts the assignments.

What is the intensity/level of danger of the problem behavior(s)?
Behavior is not dangerous but is disruptive to class and may have negative social consequences (e.g., other students have already started labeling Randall as a cry baby).

What are the events that predict when the problem behavior(s) will occur?

Related Issues (Setting Events)		Environmental Features	
___ illness	Other: ___	___ reprimand/correction	_X_ structured activity
___ drug use	_____	___ physical demands	___ unstructured time
___ negative social	_____	___ socially isolated	___ tasks too boring
___ conflict at home	_____	_X_ with peers	___ activity too long
___ academic failure	_____	_X_ other _writing activity_	___ tasks too difficult

What consequences are most likely to maintain the problem behavior(s)?

Things That Are Obtained		Things Avoided or Escaped From	
_X_ adult attention	Other: _____	___ hard tasks	Other: _____
_X_ peer attention	_____	___ reprimands	_____
___ preferred activity	_____	___ peer negatives	_____
___ money/things	_____	___ physical effort	_____

SUMMARY OF BEHAVIOR

Identify the summary that will be used to build a plan of behavior support

Setting Events and Predictors	Problem Behavior(s)	Maintaining Consequence(s)
Classes requiring written work (e.g., Social Studies, English)	Randall cries, crosses arms, puts head down, and refuses to do work	Consoling from friends, teachers, and sometimes counselor

How confident are you that the Summary of Behavior is accurate?

Not very confident					Very confident
1	2	3	4	(5)	6

What current efforts have been used to control the problem behavior?

Strategies for Preventing Problem Behavior		Consequences for Problem Behavior	
___ schedule change	Other: _____	_X_ reprimand	Other: _____
___ seating change	_____	___ office referral	_____
_X_ curriculum change	_____	___ detention	_____

FACTS–Part A

Student/Grade: _Randall – 6th_   **Date:** _12/6/02_

Interviewer: _Mr. Jensen_   **Respondent(s):** _Mrs. Nielsen_

Student profile: Please identify at least three strengths or contributions the student brings to school.

Athletic, liked by peers, and good sense of humor

Problem Behavior(s): Identify problem behaviors

___ Tardy	___ Inappropriate language	_x_ Disruptive	___ Theft
___ Unresponsive	___ Fight/Physical aggression	___ Insubordination	___ Vandalism
___ Withdrawn	___ Verbal harassment	_x_ Work not done	___ Other _____
	_x_ Verbally inappropriate	___ Self-injury	

Describe problem behavior: _Randall does not complete classwork (or homework) but instead sits at his desk, looks out the window, and plays with objects. If pressed to do work, will yell, tear up things, and/or throw things._

Identifying Routines: Where, When, and With Whom Problem Behaviors Are Most Likely.

Schedule (Times)	Activity	With Whom Does Problem Occur?	Likelihood of Problem Behavior	Specific Problem Behavior
8:30–9:30	Math	Mrs. Singh	Low High 1 2 3 4 ⑤ 6	Refuses to do work
9:30–10:30	Physical Education	Mr. Woods	① 2 3 4 5 6	
10:30–11:30	Social Studies	Mrs. Nielsen	1 2 3 4 ⑤ 6	Refuses to do work
11:30–12:00	Lunch		① 2 3 4 5 6	
12:00–12:30	Homeroom	Mr. Sanchez	① 2 3 4 5 6	
12:30–1:30	English/Language Arts	Mrs. Nielsen	1 2 3 4 5 ⑥	Refuses to do work
1:30–2:30	Science	Mrs. Avila	1 2 ③ 4 5 6	Refuses to do work
2:30–3:30	Industrial Arts	Mr. Carpenter	① 2 3 4 5 6	
			1 2 3 4 5 6	

Select one to three routines for further assessment. Select routines based on (1) similarity of activities (conditions) with ratings of 4, 5, or 6 and (2) similarity of problem behavior(s). Complete the FACTS–Part B for each routine identified.

(continued)

FIGURE 6.9. Example of a completed FACTS interview: Escape-motivated behavior. The form itself is adapted with permission from March et al. (2000).

FIGURE 6.9. *(continued)*

FACTS–Part B

Student/Grade: <u>Randall – 6th</u>   Date: <u>12/6/02</u>

Interviewer: <u>Mr. Jensen</u>   Respondent(s): <u>Mrs. Nielsen</u>

Routine/Activities/Context: Which routine (only one) from the FACTS–Part A is assessed?

Routine/Activities/Context	Problem Behavior
Classes that require homework and/or lengthy class assignments.	Does not complete work, inappropriate language, throwing objects

Provide more detail about the problem behavior(s):

What does the problem behavior(s) look like?
Randall does not complete classwork (or homework) but instead sits at his desk, looks out the window, and plays with objects. If pressed to do work, he will yell, tear up things, and/or throw things.

How often does the problem behavior(s) occur?
Six to seven times a week, when homework is due or assignments are given in class that take an extensive amount of time to complete.

How long does the problem behavior(s) last when it does occur?
It can take all period to try to get Randall to do work.

What is the intensity/level of danger of the problem behavior(s)?
Behavior is dangerous when he throws objects and is disruptive to the overall flow of classroom activity.

What are the events that predict when the problem behavior(s) will occur?

Related Issues (Setting Events)		Environmental Features	
___ illness	Other: ___	___ reprimand/correction	<u>X</u> structured activity
___ drug use	_____	___ physical demands	___ unstructured time
___ negative social	_____	___ socially isolated	___ tasks too boring
___ conflict at home	_____	___ with peers	<u>X</u> activity too long
___ academic failure	_____	<u>X</u> other <u>asked to hand in homework.</u>	___ tasks too difficult

What consequences are most likely to maintain the problem behavior(s)?

Things That Are Obtained		Things Avoided or Escaped From	
<u>X</u> adult attention	Other: _____	___ hard tasks	Other: <u>structured and/or lengthy tasks</u>
<u>X</u> peer attention	_____	___ reprimands	
___ preferred activity	_____	___ peer negatives	
___ money/things	_____	___ physical effort	_____

SUMMARY OF BEHAVIOR

Identify the summary that will be used to build a plan of behavior support

Setting Events and Predictors	Problem Behavior(s)	Maintaining Consequence(s)
Instructed to do work	Refuses to do work and yells/throws objects if pressed to do work	Does not complete work Ultimately sent to office

How confident are you that the Summary of Behavior is accurate?

Not very confident					Very confident
1	2	3	4	⑤	6

What current efforts have been used to control the problem behavior?

Strategies for Preventing Problem Behavior		Consequences for Problem Behavior	
___ schedule change	Other: _____	<u>X</u> reprimand	Other: _____
___ seating change	_____	___ office referral	_____
<u>X</u> curriculum change	_____	___ detention	_____

BEP Support Plan

Name: _Randall Prima_____ Date of Support Request: _1/6/03_____ Grade: _____

Parent's Name: _Alice Prima_____ Parent's Phone No: _504.876.5432_____

Requested by: _Mrs. Nielsen (Social Studies teacher)_____

Reason for Request: __Behavior has not improved though he's been on BEP for 1 month already____

Functional Behavioral Assessment Activities

Step 1: Gather Information (Give dates of completion)

Parent Contact _1/8/03_____ Staffing _1/13/03_____ Observation (optional) __—_____
FBA Interview _1/10/03_____ Student Interview (optional) _1/10/03_____

IEP: ____Yes _X__No No. of office referrals: ___13___ No. of absences: ___6___

Step 2: Propose a Summary Statement of the Problem

What sets off the problem?	What are the problems?	Why are they happening?
Instructed to do assignment (especially written work)	Refuses to do work and yells/throws objects if pressed to do work.	Does not complete work. Ultimately sent to office and thereby gets out of class and the assignment.

Step 3: Propose Appropriate BEP Options

❏ Basic BEP   ☒ Modified BEP   ❏ Individualized Support   ❏ Other

(continued)

FIGURE 6.10. Example of a completed BEP Support Plan.

FIGURE 6.10. *(continued)*

Design Support Plan

Step 4: Conduct BEP Team Meeting to Determine Student Goal and Design Plan

Student Goal: _Randall will complete assignments in class without disruption to himself, the_
teacher, or his peers.

Additional Supports	When	Where	Who Responsible
BEP will be monitored by his football coach.	Twice daily	Gym office	Mr. Reynolds
Randall will have opportunity to earn personally meaningful rewards on daily and weekly basis after meeting BEP goals.	Daily or weekly, dependent on goal/reinforcer set by Mr. R.	Varies	Mr. Reynolds

Step 5: Conduct Review Meetings and Use Student Monitoring Form to Monitor Progress

BEP Student Monitoring Form

Student Name: _Randall_   Facilitator Name: _Mr. Reynolds_

Student Goal: _Randall will complete assignments in class without disruption to_
himself, the teacher, or his peers.

Date	Additional Supports Completed	To do next • Continue • Modify • Monitor	Student's Progress
1/20/03	Mr. Reynolds has become Randall's BEP facilitator.	Continue	It seems to have improved his consistency in turning in DPRs.
1/27/03	Randall has earned several personally meaningful reinforcers (e.g., time to be office aide, 10 minutes' free time in gym) as a result of meeting daily goal.	Modify—Increase goal to 80% of points. Gradually fade from daily reward to weekly reward.	Randall has been meeting daily goal (75% of points). Behavior is improved. Increase in assignment completion.

BEP STUDENTS WITH AN INDIVIDUALIZED EDUCATION PLAN (IEP)

As students are identified for the BEP, the BEP team may find that a large proportion of these students are receiving special education services. This is quite common. Each student receiving special education services will have an Individualized Education Plan (IEP). The BEP and IEP teams should consider the linkage between these two programs to ensure that the best interests of each student are served. The two teams should consider the following issues:

1. The BEP should not contradict the student's IEP.
2. The BEP should support the IEP.
3. If a student has an IEP goal for behavioral issues, the BEP is not adequate to address that IEP goal.

The BEP is a targeted intervention implemented at the group level. Students who are on a basic BEP go through the same program and have the same goals. In contrast, an IEP is individualized to the needs of each individual student. The IEP is typically more comprehensive than a BEP. The IEP for a student with behavioral goals may list the following types of services and strategies: (1) half-hour of anger management class per week with the school counselor, (2) desk placed in front of the classroom, nearest the teacher, (3) early dismissal between class periods, and (4) BEP intervention. In other words, the basic BEP is only one component of the IEP. It should not be used as the sole strategy for addressing the behavioral problems of a student with an IEP for behavioral issues.

Is a modified BEP with individualized goals sufficient to address an IEP behavioral goal? This question can be answered only on a case-by-case basis. The adequacy of the IEP is dependent on the needs of the child. If the behavioral needs of a child with an IEP behavioral goal are adequately addressed and reduced by a modified BEP, then it is reasonable to assume that the BEP is adequate and sufficient. This is, however, unlikely. A student who receives special education services for behavioral issues typically has complex needs that require more than a simple, targeted intervention. When a BEP is included in a student's IEP, we recommend that it be used as one part of a comprehensive plan and not as the only strategy for addressing the student's behavioral needs.

Communication between the BEP and IEP Teams

It is essential that the individuals or teams who work to resolve the behavioral issues of a student work in concert, not in conflict. At the very least, the BEP team should have access to a list of students who have an IEP for behavioral goals. Any time a student on an IEP is considered for placement on the BEP, an IEP team member for that student should be invited to the BEP team meeting. The IEP team member can communicate the BEP team's suggestions to the rest of the IEP team.

If the IEP team chooses to incorporate the BEP into the student's IEP, they must hold an IEP meeting and make the appropriate modifications. However, placement on the BEP does not always necessitate a change in the student's IEP. A student may be placed on the BEP without any changes to the IEP. In such a case, the BEP is a service that the student receives through the school, but it is not a required part of the student's IEP contract. Placement on the BEP necessitates a change in the IEP only if (1) participation in the BEP precludes participation in some other aspect of the student's current IEP; (2) participation in the BEP creates a change in the student's IEP behavioral goals; or (3) the IEP team chooses to list the BEP as one strategy for addressing the student's IEP goal.

To enhance communication between the BEP team and special education team, we strongly suggest that the BEP team include at least one special education teacher. This teacher will attend BEP meetings as well as special education team meetings. When a student comes up for discussion with either group, the special education teacher can act as representative, communicating information between both teams.

Communication between the BEP team and special education team can be further enhanced by using the following strategies:

1. Keep a copy of the student's IEP face page in his or her BEP file. Thus, if a student comes up for "priority" discussion, the BEP team will have easy access to relevant IEP information.
2. If a student is slated for "priority" discussion at the BEP team meeting, invite the student's special education case manager to the meeting.
3. If a BEP student has an upcoming IEP meeting, invite a BEP team member to attend the meeting to share information on the student's BEP goals and progress. If the person is unable to attend, ensure lines of communication so that the IEP team can have easy access to the student's IEP data.

REMOVING A STUDENT FROM THE BEP

The BEP team may be tempted to leave a student on the BEP, indefinitely, even after a student has demonstrated consistent, significant improvement in behavior. The team may worry that the student's behavior will regress if he or she does not receive the continued support of the BEP. Keeping each student on the BEP until the end of the academic year becomes the default option for many schools. This approach can, however, unnecessarily overtax the BEP team.

For middle schools, we recommend that the BEP roster consist of no more than 30 students. Beyond 30 students, it becomes difficult to effectively manage the program and respond to issues that arise. For elementary school, we recommend a maximum of 15–20 students. Elementary school students often need more prompting, or the coordinator needs to check in and check out with the students in their classrooms. It is more time-intensive for the elementary school BEP coordinator to manage the program than it is at the middle school level. Removing students from the BEP intervention once their behavior improvements are sustainable increases the efficiency of the BEP system and is a wise use of resources. At the same time, the team must avoid removing a student whose behavior would deteriorate without the support that the BEP provides.

How does the BEP team determine when a student is ready to be faded from the BEP system? The team should begin by looking at the BEP data. We recommend that the BEP team consider removing students from the BEP on a monthly or quarterly basis. If this is a regularly occurring agenda item, there will be fewer tendencies to maintain students on a program that they no longer need.

The BEP coordinator will bring the BEP graphs, as usual, to the meeting. These graphs can be printed to show a student's data over a few days or several weeks. For this meeting, graphs should include long-term data. Prior to the meeting, the coordinator can go through the graphs and identify students who have consistently met their BEP goals (at least 80% of possible points) for at least 4 weeks. These students have demonstrated a consistent pattern of desired behavior and may be ready to maintain their behavior without the support of the BEP. The BEP coordinator can circle the graphs of each of these students, and provide copies for each BEP team member. Figure 6.11 provides an example of student data that might indicate that a student is ready to be removed from the BEP.

As a team, the group should discuss each possible candidate. The team can raise any concerns they may have about removing an individual from the BEP. A team member may have information about a student that persuades the team that the student will be unable to maintain behavioral gains without the BEP. Alternatively, the BEP may be written into a student's IEP behavioral goals. In this case, the student cannot be removed from the BEP program unless an IEP meeting is convened and the IEP team agrees that the BEP should be removed and the IEP should be changed.

If the team decides to remove a student from the BEP, they should initiate a gradual fading process rather than an immediate termination of the program for the student. For maximum effectiveness, we recommend incorporating a self-management component to scaffold the student's appropriate behavior as BEP support is faded.

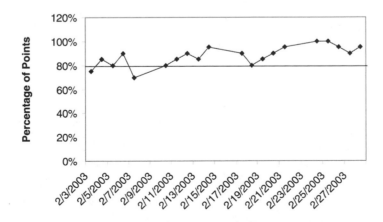

FIGURE 6.11. BEP data: Removing a student from the BEP program.

Using Self-Management to Fade BEP Support

The goal of self-management is to increase the student's sense of responsibility and ability to manage his or her own behavior without the need for redirection, prompting, and management by an adult figure. Self-management should be introduced before BEP support is faded. Self-management strategies have been described in detail in multiple publications.

We suggest that the self-management component look similar to the DPR. The goal is to shift from teacher ratings of the student's behavior to student ratings of his or her own behavior. Initially, the student and teacher will rate the student's behavior simultaneously. Each person will have his or her own copy of the DPR. At the end of the class period, the teacher and student should compare behavior ratings. At this point, the student is learning to rate his or her own behavior. Success is defined as a match between the student's score and the teacher's score. If there is a discrepancy between the two scores, the teacher and student should discuss the discrepancy and the reason for the teacher's decision. The teacher's score is assumed to be the accurate score. The emphasis of this first stage is for the student's ratings to come closer and closer to approximating the teacher's ratings, until the student is reliably and accurately rating his or her own behavior.

In order to encourage the student's reliability, the student can earn small rewards for having the same score as the teacher. For example, if a student gives him- or herself a rating of 1, 1, 1, 2 on the four behavior goals, and the teacher gives the same rating, the student could earn a High 5. Typically, this would be discouraged because the student should not earn a High 5 for suboptimal behavior. In the early stages of BEP removal, however, the student earns rewards for accuracy and honesty rather than for behavior.

Once the student can rate his or her behavior reliably, rewards for accuracy can be faded, and rewards for appropriate behavior can be reinstated. The next goal is to remove the teacher-rating component. The number of times that the teacher provides a rating is gradually reduced. For example, during the first week of BEP removal, the teacher will provide a rating on 4 of 5 days. The student rating is used once. In the next week, the teacher provides ratings on 3 days.

In addition to fading teacher ratings, the student's participation in the check-in/check-out system can be faded as well. While the student is learning to self-assess his or her own behavior, he or she continues to check in and check out and to turn in a DPR. The BEP coordinator continues to collect, enter, and analyze the student's BEP data during the time that he or she is learning to rate his or her own behavior. Data collection at this point is critical. The BEP data will demonstrate whether the student's behavior stays the same, improves, or significantly worsens, as the BEP is gradually faded. In the case of worsening behavior, the team should discuss whether or not the student is ready to move to self-management. The worsening behavior may be an indication that it is too early to remove the BEP support. Alternatively, it may be an indication that the BEP fading process has not been adequately explained to the student, or effectively implemented.

A clear conversation between the student and an adult regarding the goals and process of the self-management strategy is critical to its success. Any member of the BEP team may lead this discussion with the student. We recommend using someone who knows the student well and whom the student views as actively involved in the BEP process. During this discussion, the adult should explain to the student that he or she is pleased with the student's behavioral improvements and believes the student has demonstrated maturity and a readiness to be responsible for his or her own behavior. The adult should share a copy of the student's data with him or her. These data should already be familiar to the student, but the emphasis in this conversation is to demonstrate the student's consistent performance above the 80% goal. The adult should then explain that the student's accomplishment will be recognized by allowing the student to become a self-manager, without need for the BEP. Finally, the adult should explain what the student can expect as the BEP system is gradually faded. The adult should have the student practice using the self-management card several times. The student should leave this meeting feeling a sense of pride and accomplishment in his or her behavioral accomplishments as well as motivation to continue to demonstrate appropriate behavior.

The BEP coordinator should talk with the student's parent(s) and explain the reason for removing the student from the BEP. The counselor or BEP member should emphasize ways that the parent(s) can continue to support and encourage the student's appropriate behavior.

What If the Student Wants to Stay on the BEP System?

We have found that, in schools where the BEP system is running well, students like being on the BEP. Students view the program positively. A student may view BEP removal as a punishment rather than as a recognition or promotion. The student may, in fact, respond by increasing his or her inappropriate behavior.

If a middle school student wants to stay on the BEP, there is no reason why he or she cannot continue to check in and check out. At the middle school level, this will not pose an unnecessary burden on the resources of the BEP team. Because the student continues to rate him- or herself on the DPR, the teacher's time is not unnecessarily spent. Also, although the student continues to check in and check out, the BEP team no longer enters, analyzes, or responds to the data. They simply file the student's DPR in the student's folder. The student can continue to have daily contact with a person he or she enjoys without creating any additional workload for the BEP team. This makes it possible for a new student to begin the BEP in his or her place.

7

Frequently Asked Questions about Implementation of the BEP

Implementing the BEP is relatively straightforward and takes little staff time. There are, however, common issues that have come up in schools that have instituted this program. The purpose of this chapter is to address frequently asked questions regarding establishing the BEP system of support.

WHAT IF A STUDENT DOES NOT CHECK IN IN THE MORNING?

One of the first questions schools ask is what to do if students are not checking in on a regular basis. Part of the duties of the BEP coordinator will be to determine if students on the BEP are absent or have merely forgotten to check in in the morning. If a student has just forgotten to check in, the BEP coordinator delivers the DPR to the student and prompts him or her to try to remember to check in the next day. Although the BEP coordinator should not make a habit of delivering DPRs to students, if a student forgot to get the form, he or she should not miss out on opportunities for feedback and to meet his or her daily point goal. After all, this is a system to increase positive feedback and success of students at risk for severe problem behavior.

WHAT IF A STUDENT DOES NOT CHECK OUT IN THE AFTERNOON?

In some cases the student will not check out but will bring the DPR back with him or her the following morning, in many cases signed by the parent or caregiver. It is at that time that the BEP coordinator can prompt the student to check out that day. Also, it is important to record the information from the DPR into the BEP database. The student may have met his or her goal but forgot to check out. You do not want to penalize the student (or give a "0" for the day) to a student who forgot to check out.

There will be times that the student does not check out, nor bring the card back the next day. In this case, the student receives a "0" for that day. The BEP coordinator should ask the student why he or she did not check out and prompt him or her to remember to check out that day. Teachers can also play a role in reminding students to check out by prompting them toward the end of the school day (e.g., "Kiran, remember to check out when the bell rings."). This prompting from teachers should be faded over time so that students can become independent in participating in the program. For younger students, the prompting may need to occur for a longer period of time.

WHAT IF A STUDENT IS *CONSISTENTLY* NOT CHECKING IN OR CHECKING OUT?

The BEP coordinator should sit down with the student and determine what barriers are preventing him or her from checking in or out. For example, one student we worked with was not checking out after school because he would miss his bus if he did. To resolve this issue the BEP coordinator spoke with his sixth-period teacher, and she agreed that the student could leave 5 minutes early from class to check out at the end of the day. Some students may say, "I forgot to check in or check out." There are several solutions that can be tried. Enlist the help of the student's friends to remind him or her to check in and check out. Simple statements such as "Hey, can you do me a favor? Can you help your buddy Sean remember to check in in the mornings?" by the BEP coordinator often work. It is a good idea to reinforce the buddy you have enlisted for helping the student on the BEP. Another suggestion is to go to the student's last class and escort him or her to check out for several days in a week to provide the student with practice with this behavior. Remember, some of the students are on the BEP due to poor organization skills and may need extra practice learning a new routine.

Some students may not check out because they have had a bad day and have not met their behavioral goal. There should be an incentive for checking out, even if the student has not met his or her goal. For example, the raffle system mentioned earlier, in which students received a BEP raffle ticket just for checking in or checking out, is effective. The raffle was held once a week, and only students on the BEP were eligible. The more times a student checked in and checked out, the more tickets he or she had and the more chances to win. Raffle prizes were small and inexpensive, consisting mainly of small treats, pencils, or small toys.

When troubleshooting why students are not consistently checking in and out, it is important to determine whether the student has "bought in" to the program and is voluntarily participating. There have been times when a parent wants the student on the BEP but the student resists by not following through with the program requirements. Remember this is a voluntary, positive support system. Efforts should be made to find reinforcers that are meaningful for students who have not bought in to the program. One student we worked with was having difficulty meeting the requirements of the BEP, but was interested in earning a baseball hat rather than receiving daily rewards. An individual contract was developed for this student so that after a certain number of weeks of meeting his goal he would be able to earn the hat. There will be times when students refuse to participate no matter what adaptations are made, and for these students more individualized, intensive assessment and intervention are likely necessary

The location of where students check in and check out is critical. It needs to be a place students can easily access as well as one that is separated from the loud disruption of common areas such as hallways and cafeterias. In some schools where we have seen inconsistency in students checking in and out, either the location was inconvenient (i.e., not centrally located) or there had not been a permanent place set up for the process. For example, one of the schools we worked in chose the library as a check-in/check-out location. This location usually worked well, but was not available at times when parent groups met in the library after school, which disrupted the check-out process.

Although the check-in/check-out location needs to be in a quiet area, it does help if it is located near a common area so that the BEP coordinator can scan the area to look for students who have not checked in. It is important to build independence in the process of participating in the BEP, but is also helps to provide prompts to students who may need them. In middle schools, in particular, students are heavily invested in peer interaction. It may take some prompting to help break them away from their peers to check in.

WHAT IF *SEVERAL* STUDENTS ARE NOT CHECKING IN AND OUT?

If several students are not checking in and out, the implementation of the whole intervention needs to be examined. One question that should be answered is *Has the school given the BEP a high profile?* Elsewhere in this manual we describe how to give the BEP a high profile and ensure that it is a positive intervention. Without that boost, the BEP may be seen as just another educational innovation that will pass with time. In one of the schools we worked with, the staff were not well trained on how to implement the intervention. There was disagreement as to which students should be placed on the BEP, and issues were raised about existing programs that interfered or overlapped with the BEP. In that school, there were some staff who were "sabotaging" the intervention. That is, since the staff members were not in agreement with how the BEP should be implemented and with whom, they did not put much effort into the intervention and were not providing students with regular feedback. From this experience we have learned that schools should complete the Implementation Readiness Questionnaire (see Appendix K) and have staff buy in to the program prior to implementing this system of support.

Another question to answer if many students are not checking in and out is *Is the BEP coordinator a person whom students enjoy and look forward to interacting with?* In some of the schools in which we have worked, the BEP coordinator is chosen based on time availability, rather than on his or her personality "fit" with the students. Although educators typically go into the business of working in schools because they enjoy working with children, there are usually teachers or paraprofessionals that the students really resonate with, enjoy being around, and will work hard for. In one of the middle schools we worked in, the BEP coordinator had an art of joking with students to improve their moods or reduce tension. These students could not wait to interact with her on a daily basis, and she was often sought out for problem solving with other staff around student issues.

In another school we worked in, the BEP coordinator was a paraprofessional who was placed in the position out of default: She was available before and after school. Although she was very effective in supporting teachers, she did not really want the job as BEP coordinator, and this came through in her interactions with students. She was often short with them, more negative than positive, and had a hard time managing the numbers of students who were checking in and out daily. She would complain in front of students that she did not like the BEP. It is easy to see why, over time, students would not want to engage in the BEP intervention in this situation.

WHAT IF THE STUDENT LOSES HIS OR HER BEP DAILY PROGRESS REPORT?

One of the responsibilities for the student on the BEP includes carrying the DPR from class to class, teacher to teacher, or, in the case of elementary school students, from setting to setting. We recommend teaching the students to get another DPR as soon as they realize they have lost it. That way, although they may have lost some points toward their goal by losing the DPR, they have not lost their points for the entire day. They can receive feedback on their new DPR and continue to receive positive feedback throughout the day. For younger students, some may need the DPR to be placed on a clipboard so that it is less likely to get lost during transitions.

Students may also lose DPR cards if they find that being on the BEP is not helpful or rewarding. For those students, troubleshoot ways to improve the program. Often this involves asking them the types of rewards they are interested in working for (e.g., baseball cap). Some students may "lose" their DPR if they have had a bad day and are afraid to bring the DPR home to their parents. As sad as it may be, there have been parents who punish students severely for having a "bad day" at school. In these situations we have either encouraged the parents to use the program positively, or we have had students not take their cards home as part of the program. We cannot overemphasize that the BEP needs to be a positive program, one the students enjoy participating in. If the student gets into even more trouble by being on the BEP, he or she is going to be less likely to participate.

WHAT IF STAFF ARE NOT IMPLEMENTING THE BEP CORRECTLY?

All staff should receive in-service training on the purpose of the BEP, the positive nature of the program, and how to provide feedback to students. At times, teachers will write negative comments on the DPR, or some teachers may use it as a tool to punish students by writing all of the inappropriate behaviors the students engaged in on the form. Some teachers may need individual training and follow-up to reemphasize the positive nature of the program and to provide prompts for positive feedback. Many schools we have worked with have a line for teacher feedback on the DPR that prompts them to write positive rather than negative comments. For example, one school we worked with had a school-wide positive reinforcement system in which students would receive "Wow!" tickets for following school-wide expectations. In this school, the word "Wow!" was written next to the line for additional teacher feedback on the DPR (see Appendix D). This provided teachers with a visual prompt for positive feedback and was consistent with school-wide acknowledgment systems.

One way to keep the system positive and teachers invested is to make sure they are receiving feedback, at least quarterly, on how students on the BEP are doing. One thing that happens frequently in schools is that the teacher helps in the data collection process (i.e., filling out office discipline referral forms for students engaging in severe or dangerous behavior or completing the DPR), but never sees a summary of the data or how they are used to make decisions in schools. Staff should be updated on how many students are served on the BEP, how many are meeting their goals on a regular basis, and other outcome data associated with BEP improvements (e.g., student improvements in grades and test scores).

To keep the system positive, a school may also want to reward staff on a frequent basis for their participation in the BEP. For example, staff are required to initial DPRs for students participating in the BEP and are asked to write positive comments when appropriate. Teacher's names could be randomly selected from the student DPRs at monthly staff meetings to earn small prizes, or prizes could be given for the most creative or encouraging comments written on student DPRs. Students on the BEP could also nominate staff that they thought helped them be successful on the BEP. This person could be recognized at a faculty meeting, assembly, or in the school newsletter.

WHAT IF PARENTS OR CAREGIVERS ARE NOT FOLLOWING THROUGH OR USE THE BEP AS A PUNITIVE SYSTEM?

One of the strengths of the BEP is the increased connection between home and school. Parents and caregivers are given daily feedback on how their student is doing in school. In some cases, we have had difficulty getting parents to follow through with reviewing the DPR nightly and providing positive feedback to the student. In these cases, we may call or meet with the parents to emphasize the importance of their participation. Many of the schools that we work with have parents, school staff, and students sign a "BEP Contract" agreeing to the responsibilities of participating in the BEP. This provides parents with clear expectations for the program and can be referred to to remind parents of their responsibilities.

One interesting finding gleaned from our research is that the parent element of the BEP tends to be the weakest element when examining fidelity of BEP implementation. Results from Hawken and Horner (in press) indicate that four of the critical features of the BEP (i.e., students checking in, regular teacher feedback, students checking out, and daily DPR data used for decision making) were implemented with an average of 87% fidelity across students. Parental feedback (i.e., signature on the DPR) was provided during only 67% of the fidelity of implementation checks. It should be noted, however, that many of the students were successful on the BEP and were meeting daily point goals despite lack of parental participation. In essence, parental feedback is encouraged but not necessary for student success on the BEP. There are many students who could benefit from the BEP who come from chaotic home environments. These students should be given equal opportunity to benefit from the BEP even if their parents are unable to participate. (Note: Parents should still give permission for the student to participate in the BEP.)

There are unfortunate circumstances we have come across in schools in which students participating in the BEP are punished for having "bad days." A bad day may mean that the student has not met his or her goal for that day. Some parents have implemented harsh punishments (e.g., spanking, hitting, yelling, extreme limitation of activities) when the DPR was brought home and the student had not done as well as expected. We typically hear about this from the student, or the student stops wanting to participate in the BEP. In these instances, we have set up "surrogate parents" at the school who serve as the additional person who provides feedback, praise, and comments on the DPR. The surrogate parent could be a teacher (other than the student's regular teacher), custodian, paraprofessional, volunteer who is in the school daily, or some other adult who can commit 5 minutes each day to reviewing the student's DPR and providing positive feedback. The issue of harsh punishment will need to be addressed with the parent and would probably be best handled by having either the counselor, principal, or vice principal meet with the parent.

WHAT IF A STUDENT IS CONSISTENTLY PARTICIPATING IN THE BEP AND HIS OR HER BEHAVIOR GETS WORSE?

It is expected that within about 2 weeks, students' behavior should improve on the BEP. For students who are receiving support to improve academic outcomes, it may take longer to notice changes in grades, but there should be an increase in organization, homework completion, and the like. Students whose behavior gets worse may need a more intensive, individualized intervention. Additional assessment data can be taken using functional behavioral assessment procedures. It is likely that classroom observations will be included when gathering information. Once information is gathered, it is used to develop an individualized behavior support plan. For more information on Functional Behavioral Assessment and Behavior Support Planning, see Crone and Horner (2003).

Appendices

List of Acronyms and Definitions

BEP. Behavior Education Program. The BEP is a daily check-in/check-out system that provides the student with immediate feedback on his or her behavior (via teacher rating on a Daily Progress Report) and increased positive adult attention.

BSP. Behavior Support Plan. An individualized plan to address a student's behavioral goals and objectives. The BSP should describe the intervention strategies to be used, the person responsible for implementation, a timeline for implementation, and the means by which the outcomes of the BSP will be evaluated.

DPR. Daily Progress Report. The DPR is the form used in the Behavior Education Program to track a student's daily progress towards meeting his or her behavioral goals. Samples of several DPRs are provided in the Appendices.

ELL. English Language Learner. An ELL student is a student whose native language is not English. ELL students are often provided with language support and instruction through placement in ELL classrooms or programs.

FBA. Functional Behavioral Assessment. An assessment of a person's behavior that is based on determining the function that the behavior serves for that person. The assessment typically consists of interviews with teachers, the student, and parents, as well as observations of the student's behavior in the problematic setting. The information gained from the FBA is used to develop a hypothesis regarding the purpose of the student's behavior and the circumstances under which the behavior occurs. The assessment information is used to build an individualized behavior support plan for that student.

IEP. Individualized Education Plan. An IEP describes the educational program that has been designed to meet the needs of any student who receives special education and related services. Each IEP should be a truly individualized document. The document identifies the student's needs, goals, and objectives, and strategies that will be implemented in the school to meet those objectives. Frequency and duration of the strategies should be included as well.

APPENDIX B

Request for Assistance Form

Date _____   Teacher/Team _____
                             IEP: Yes No (Circle)
Student Name _____   Grade _____

Situations	Problem Behaviors	Most Common Result
What have you tried/used? How has it worked? Why do you think the behavior keeps happening?		

What is your behavioral goal/expectation for this student?   _____

What have you tried to date to change the situations in which the problem behavior(s) occur?

__ Modified assignments to match the student's skills	__ Changed seating assignments	__ Changed schedule of activities	Other?
__ Arranged tutoring to improve the student's academic skills	__ Changed curriculum	__ Provided extra assistance	

What have you tried to date to teach expected behaviors?

__ Reminders about expected behavior when problem behavior is likely	__ Clarified rules and expected behavior for the whole class	__ Practiced the expected behaviors in class	Other?
__ Reward program for expected behavior	__ Oral agreement with the student	__ Self-management program	
__ Systematic feedback about behavior	__ Individual written contract with the student	__ Contract with student/ with parents	

What consequences have you tried to date for the problem behavior?

__ Loss of privileges	__ Note or phone call to the student's parents	__ Office referral	Other?
__ Time-out	__ Detention	__ Reprimand	
__ Referral to school counselor	__ Meeting with the student's parents	__ Individual meeting with the student	

From Todd, Horner, Sugai, and Colvin (1999). Copyright 1999 by Lawrence Erlbaum Associates. Reprinted by permission.

Daily Progress Report—Middle School, Example 1

A- Day   B-Day

Name:_____   Date:_____

Teachers: Please indicate YES (2), So-So (1), or No (0) regarding the student's achievement for the following goals.

Goals	1/5			2/6			3/7			HR			4/8		
Be respectful	2	1	0	2	1	0	2	1	0	2	1	0	2	1	0
Be responsible	2	1	0	2	1	0	2	1	0	2	1	0	2	1	0
Keep Hands and Feet to Self	2	1	0	2	1	0	2	1	0	2	1	0	2	1	0
Follow Directions	2	1	0	2	1	0	2	1	0	2	1	0	2	1	0
Be There – Be Ready	2	1	0	2	1	0	2	1	0	2	1	0	2	1	0
TOTAL POINTS															
TEACHER INITIALS															

BEP Daily Goal /   50   BEP Daily Score   /50

In training_____   BEP Member_____   _____
                                                            Student signature

Teacher comments: Please state briefly any specific behaviors or achievements that demonstrate the student's progress. (If additional space is required, please attach a note and indicate so below)

Period 1/5_____

Period 2/6_____

Period 3/7_____

Home Room_____

Period 4/8_____

Parent/Caregiver Signature: _____

Parent/Caregiver Comments: _____

Daily Progress Report—Middle School, Example 2

Name _____

	Materials To Class	Worked and Let Others Work	Follow Directions the First Time		Teacher	Parent
	2 1 No	2 1 No	2 1 No	Assignments:		
				Wow,		
	2 1 No	2 1 No	2 1 No	Assignments:		
				Wow,		
	2 1 No	2 1 No	2 1 No	Assignments:		
				Wow,		
	2 1 No	2 1 No	2 1 No	Assignments:		
				Wow,		
	2 1 No	2 1 No	2 1 No	Assignments:		
				Wow,		

High-5 Ticket

```
┌─────────────────────────────────────────────────────┐
│                                                       │
│                   HIGH-5 TICKET                       │
│                                                       │
│                                                       │
│   Student Name: _____         │
│                                                       │
│                                                       │
│   Issued by: _____          │
│                                                       │
│                                                       │
│   Date: _____          │
│                                                       │
│                                                       │
│                 KEEP THE POWER!                       │
│                                                       │
└─────────────────────────────────────────────────────┘
```

From Fern Ridge Middle School (1999). Reprinted with permission from the authors.

Daily Progress Report—Elementary School, Example 1

Name: _____

Date: _____

2 = Good

1 = Needs work

Points earned: _____

Goal: _____ Goal reached? Yes No

GOALS	Reading	Math	Lunch	Recess	Music	Art	Library	PE	Title I
Play Safe									
Act Fair									
Work Hard									
Total Points									

Teacher Comments: _____

_____

Parent Comments: _____

_____

Parent/Guardian Signature: _____

Please sign and have your child return this form on a daily basis!

Daily Progress Report—Elementary School, Example 2

Name: _____

Date: _____

RATING SCALE
3 = Great
2 = "Sorta"
1 = Try again

Points possible _____
Points received _____
% of points _____
Goal met?   Yes   No

GOALS:	Morning work	Reading	Math	PE/Music	Spelling/Writing	Resource	Afternoon
1.							
2.							
3.							

COMMENTS: _____
_____
_____
_____

99

Daily Progress Report—Elementary School, Example 3

Name: _____

Date: _____

= 2 points

= 1 point

= 0 points

Points received _____

Points possible _____

Daily goal reached?   Yes   No

GOALS	Morning	PE/Music	Reading	Math	Afternoon
	😊 😊 😊	😊 😊 😊	😊 😊 😊	😊 😊 😊	😊 😊 😊
	😊 😊 😊	😊 😊 😊	😊 😊 😊	😊 😊 😊	😊 😊 😊
	😊 😊 😊	😊 😊 😊	😊 😊 😊	😊 😊 😊	😊 😊 😊

From Deanne A. Crone, Robert H. Horner, and Leanne S. Hawken (2004). Copyright by The Guilford Press. Permission to photocopy this appendix is granted to purchasers of this book for personal use only (see copyright page for details).

BEP $1.00 Coupon

$$$	BEP Coupon	$$$
	1	
Good for $1.00 at School Store		Principal Signature _____
$$$	BEP Coupon	$$$

From Fern Ridge Middle School (1999). Reprinted with permission from the authors.

Working Smarter, Not Harder

Committee, project, or initiative	Purpose	Outcome	Target group	Staff involved

Reprinted with permission from George Sugai.

BEP Implementation Readiness Questionnaire

Is your school ready to implement the BEP? Prior to implementation, it is recommended that the following features be in place. Please circle the answer that best describes your school at this time.

Yes   No   1. Our school has a school-wide discipline system in place. In essence, we have decided on three to five rules, taught the rules to students, provide rewards to students for following the rules and provide mild consequences for rule infractions.

Yes   No   2. We have secured staff "buy in" for implementation of the BEP. In essence, the staff agrees that this is an intervention needed in the school to support students at risk for more severe forms of problem behavior.

Yes   No   3. There is administrative support for implementation of the BEP intervention. In essence, there is money allocated for the implementation of the program.

Yes   No   4. There have been no major changes in the school system that would prevent successful implementation of the BEP intervention. Major changes include things such as teacher strikes, high teacher or administrative turnover, or major changes in funding.

Yes   No   5. We have made implementation of the BEP one of our top three priorities for this school year.

BEP Check-In and Check-Out Record

Date: _____   BEP coordinator: _____

| | Check-In | | | | | Check-Out |
Student name	Paper	Pencil	Notebook	BEP Parent Copy		BEP School Copy

BEP Team Meeting Agenda

Date: _____   Note taker: _____

Team Members Present: _____

List of Priority Students:

1. Discuss priority students.

2. Discuss new referrals.

3. Identify students to receive $1.00 school store coupon.

4. Other BEP issues or students.

"Priority Student" Decision Sheet

1. Look at BEP graphs.

2. Look at office discipline referral reports.

3. What subjective information do you have about the student from this week that adds to our understanding of the student?

4. Make one of four decisions.

   - Student is ready to be removed from BEP.

   - Things are going fine; keep on current BEP.

   - Having some problems—think of simple additional supports. (Who is responsible? Timeline?)

   - Having larger problem—student needs a comprehensive, function-based assessment and intervention. (Who is responsible? Timeline?)

BEP Team Action Plan

Date: _____ Student: _____(Initials only)

Action Plan item: _____

Discussion:

Task	Person Responsible	Date to be Completed	Comments

Action Plan item: _____

Discussion:

Task	Person Responsible	Date to be Completed	Comments

BEP Contract

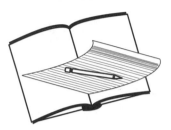

I, _____ , agree to work on these things this year.

1. _____

2. _____

3. _____

I will work with _____ to keep track of my progress. I understand that I will have a chance to earn a reward each week when I meet my goals. A list of rewards I would like to earn include:

1. _____

2. _____

3. _____

I will try hard to do my best to meet these goals every day.

_____
Signature of Student

I will do my best to help _____ meet his/her goals every day.

_____   _____
Signature of Coordinator   Signature of Parent

BEP Support Plan

Name: _____ Date of Support Request: _____ Grade: _____

Parent's Name: _____ Parent's Phone No: _____

Requested by: _____

Reason for Request: _____

Functional Behavioral Assessment Activities

Step 1: Gather Information (Give dates of completion)

Parent Contact _____ Staffing _____ Observation (optional) _____
FBA Interview _____ Student Interview (optional) _____

IEP: ____Yes ____No   No. of office referrals: _____   No. of absences: _____

Step 2: Propose a Summary Statement of the Problem

What sets off the problem?	What are the problems?	Why are they happening?

Step 3: Propose Appropriate BEP Options

❑ Basic BEP   ❑ Modified BEP   ❑ Individualized Support   ❑ Other

(continued)

Design Support Plan

Step 4: Conduct BEP Team Meeting to Determine Student Goal and Design Plan

Student Goal: _____

_____

Additional Supports	When	Where	Who Responsible

Step 5: Conduct Review Meetings and Use Student Monitoring Form to Monitor Progress

BEP Student Monitoring Form

Student Name: _____ Facilitator Name: _____

Student Goal: _____

_____

Date	Additional Supports Completed	To do next • Continue • Modify • Monitor	Student's Progress

Functional Behavioral Assessment–Behavior Support Plan Protocol (F-BSP Protocol)

FUNCTIONAL BEHAVIORAL ASSESSMENT INTERVIEW—TEACHER/STAFF/PARENT

Student Name: _____ Age: _____ Grade: _____ Date: _____

Person(s) interviewed: _____

Interviewer: _____

Student Profile: What is the student good at or what are some strengths that the student brings to school?

_____

_____

Step 1A: Interview Teacher/Staff/Parent

Description of the Behavior

What does the problem behavior(s) look like?
How often does the problem behavior(s) occur?
How long does the problem behavior(s) last when it does occur?
How disruptive or dangerous is the problem behavior(s)?

Description of the Antecedent
Identifying Routines: When, where, and with whom are problem behaviors most likely?

Schedule (Times)	Activity	Specific Problem Behavior	Likelihood of Problem Behavior	With Whom Does Problem Occur?
			Low High 1 2 3 4 5 6	
			1 2 3 4 5 6	
			1 2 3 4 5 6	
			1 2 3 4 5 6	
			1 2 3 4 5 6	
			1 2 3 4 5 6	
			1 2 3 4 5 6	
			1 2 3 4 5 6	

(continued)

Summarize Antecedent (and Setting Events)

What situations seem to set off the problem behavior? (difficult tasks, transitions, structured activities, small-group settings, teacher's request, particular individuals, etc.)

When is the problem behavior most likely to occur? (times of day and days of the week)

When is the problem behavior least likely to occur? (times of day and days of the week)

Setting Events: Are there specific conditions, events, or activities that make the problem behavior worse? (missed medication, history of academic failure, conflict at home, missed meals, lack of sleep, history of problems with peers, etc.)

Description of the Consequence

What usually happens after the behavior occurs? (what is the teacher's reaction, how do other students react, is the student sent to the office, does the student get out of doing work, does the student get in a power struggle, etc.)

- - - - - - End of Interview - - - - - -

Step 2A: Propose a Testable Explanation

Setting Event	Antecedent	Behavior	Consequence
		1.	
		2.	

Function of the Behavior

For each ABC sequence listed above, why do you think the behavior is occurring? (to get teacher attention, peer attention, desired object/activity, or escape undesirable activity, demand, particular people, etc.)

1. _____

2. _____

How confident are you that your testable explanation is accurate?

Very sure			So-so		Not at all sure
6	5	4	3	2	1

(continued)

INSTRUCTIONS FOR COMPLETING THE FUNCTIONAL BEHAVIORAL ASSESSMENT–BEHAVIOR SUPPORT PLAN PROTOCOL (F-BSP PROTOCOL)

The F-BSP Protocol was designed as a tool to guide the process of completing a functional behavioral assessment (FBA) and of linking the assessment to the design of an individual behavior support plan (BSP). The F-BSP Protocol is divided into eight Steps: (1) Interview Teacher/Staff/Parent/Student; (2) Propose a Testable Explanation; (3) Rate Your Confidence in the Testable Explanation; (4) Conduct Observations; (5) Confirm/Modify Testable Explanation; (6) Build a Competing Behavior Pathway; (7) Select Intervention Strategies; and (8) Evaluation Plan.

The F-BSP Protocol can be used to complete either a simple FBA or a full FBA. In a simple FBA, Steps 4 and 5 are omitted. The Student Interview portion of Step 1 is omitted as well in a simple FBA.

Demographic Information

Before any interview, it is important to explain the purpose of the interview to the interviewee. Spend a little time explaining why you are doing the interview, indicate that you think it will take about 20–30 minutes to complete, and note that you will follow up with the interviewee once the FBA is completed.

Take a few minutes to complete the demographic information at the top of page 1. For confidentiality purposes, you may choose to use only the student's initials or to identify the student by his or her student number.

In the space next to "Person(s) Interviewed," indicate the person's relationship to the student, (math teacher, lunchroom monitor, parent, etc). In the space next to "Interviewer," indicate the interviewer's role in the behavior support process (Action Team member, team leader, school psychologist, etc.).

In the space next to "Student Profile," ask the interviewee to list some of the student's strengths, skills, or talents. Also list items or activities that the student enjoys or will work for. This information will help you to design a BSP that builds on the student's strengths and that includes consequences that are personally reinforcing to the student.

Step 1A: Interview Teacher/Staff/Parent

The purpose of Step 1 is to get a clear understanding of the problem behavior(s) of concern and to identify routines that predict or support the problem behavior. This is accomplished by generating a clear definition of the problem behavior, and by identifying the setting events, antecedents, and consequences of the problem behavior.

The first interview should be conducted with the person who made the initial request for assistance. This may be the student's primary teacher or any other adult with whom the student has significant contact (e.g., the lunchroom monitor, school counselor, or algebra teacher). A simple FBA typically includes only one teacher interview. A full FBA may include additional interviews with relevant adults, including other teachers or a parent. Copies of the teacher/staff/parent interview can be made to accommodate the need for multiple interviews.

(continued)

Description of the Behavior

The interviewer asks the interviewee four questions regarding the problem behavior.

1. What does the problem behavior(s) look like?
2. How often does the problem behavior(s) occur?
3. How long does the problem behavior(s) last when it does occur?
4. How disruptive or dangerous is the problem behavior?

Write down the answers to each question in the space provided. Prompt the interviewee to be as specific as possible. If the answer to the question is not specific, measurable, or observable, prompt the interviewee to be clearer in his or her response. For example, in response to question 1, the interviewee may say "*Marisa is spacey and distractible in class.*" This definition of the problem behavior is unclear— "spacey and distractible" may mean something different to the interviewer than it does to the interviewee. Prompt the interviewee by saying, "*How do you know when Marisa is being spacey and distractible? What does it look like?*" Continue to prompt the interviewee until the description of the problem behavior is clear enough that two observers would be able to recognize it independently. If the interviewee describes more than one problem behavior in question 1, be sure to get answers to questions 2, 3, and 4 for each problem behavior. Make a clear note of this on the interview form.

Description of the Antecedent

An *antecedent* is an event or circumstance that happens before a behavior occurs. It can be thought of as the predictor of a problem behavior. Examples of antecedents that could set off problem behavior include asking the student to do a demanding or long task; placing the student next to another child whom he or she dislikes; or expecting a student to complete a task during unstructured work time. The same antecedent could set off problem behavior for one student, while it helps another student to perform successfully. Because antecedents can vary so much among different students, it is very important to understand the antecedents that matter to the student with whom you are concerned. You can begin to identify the antecedents to problem behavior by looking at the student's daily routine.

Begin by completing the table on the bottom of page 1. In the first two columns, fill in the student's daily schedule. In the first column, indicate the time period for the activity, and in the second column briefly describe the activity. For example, for a middle school student you would write down the time for first period and the name of the class that the student has during first period. Then you would continue on through the last period of the day. The schedule for an elementary school student can be obtained from the student's primary teacher. An elementary school schedule is usually broken into smaller time periods, by subject or activity (e.g., math, science, circle time, etc.). The interview will go quicker if you can get the child's schedule and complete this section before you begin the interview. If you are interviewing a parent, you will complete the first two columns of this table a little differently. Ask the parent to think of the times of their day that are related to school. Some examples include getting ready for school in the morning, transportation to school, transportation home from school, and doing homework. Include all of these activities in the "Activity" column. Ask the parent to provide you with a general idea of times when these activities occur.

Complete the rest of the table for the time periods you have listed. Look at the first time period. Ask the interviewee if the student engages in problem behavior during that time period. If he or she does, ask the interviewee what type of problem behavior occurs. Write this down in the column marked "Specific Problem Behavior." The problem behaviors that you write down should reflect the problem behaviors that you discussed in the first section of the interview. You should already have a good description of these behaviors, so it is fine to write a brief description in this column (e.g., you could write "temper tantrum," "fighting," or "distractible" because these behaviors are specifically described in the first section).

(continued)

After you have written down the type of problem behavior that occurs during a time period, ask the interviewee how likely it is that the problem behavior will occur during that time period. Ask him or her to rate the likelihood on a scale of 1 to 6, where 1 means that it rarely happens and 6 means that it happens on a daily basis. Circle that number in the next column.

Finally, ask the interviewee with whom the problem is most likely to occur. Does the student get into trouble with other students? Is the student defiant toward the teacher? Perhaps the problem does not impact anyone other than the student. In this column, indicate if the problem occurs with peers, teacher, self, parent, or another significant person. If the interviewee indicates that the problem typically occurs with specific peers, you should indicate these students by using their initials only. Complete each of these columns for each time period listed.

Summarize Antecedent (and Setting Events)

The next section helps you to summarize and clarify the information you have learned from the description of the student's schedule. In this section, the interviewee will answer four questions:

1. What situations seem to set off the problem behavior?
2. When is the problem behavior most likely to occur?
3. When is the problem behavior least likely to occur?
4. Are there specific conditions, events, or activities that make the problem behavior worse?

To answer the first question, take a look at the completed table with the interviewee. First look at the times when the student is most likely to engage in problem behavior—times when the likelihood is rated a 4, 5, or 6. Is there anything similar about those times? For example, is each time period an unstructured time, or do each of the time periods require the student to do demanding work on his or her own? Perhaps each is a time when the student's sibling is in the same class. Try to determine what is similar about the problematic routines that tend to set off the problem behavior. If the interviewee has trouble answering this question, prompt him or her by saying "*If you wanted to make the problem behavior occur, what would you do?*"

Ask the interviewee what times of the day and days of the week the problem behavior is most likely to occur. If his or her answer is different than what you would expect (based on the information given in the schedule table), ask the interviewee to clarify his or her answer.

Ask the interviewee when the problem behavior is least likely to occur. Knowing when the problem behavior does not occur can help you identify things that work for the student. That is, there are some routines when the student does not get into trouble. If you can identify what it is about those routines that helps the student be successful, you can better determine how to change the student's unsuccessful routines.

Setting events are situations or circumstances that make it more likely that a problem behavior will occur or that make the problem behavior more intense. Some examples include: if the student has a fight with a parent right before coming to school, if the student didn't get enough sleep or missed a meal, or if the student misses taking medication. Ask the interviewee if he or she knows of certain situations that tend to make the student's problem behavior worse, or more likely to occur.

Description of the Consequence

In this section, you want to find out what usually happens after the problem behavior occurs. Is the student ignored or do all of his peers start to laugh? Is the student sent to the office? Is the student sent to time-out? Ask the interviewee what typically happens after the problem behavior occurs and what impact those consequences seem to have on the problem behavior. In other words, do the consequences make the problem behavior stop, improve, or get worse?

(continued)

End of Interview

At this point, the face-to-face portion of the interview is completed. Next you will summarize the information you have learned from the interview to create a "testable explanation" of why the problem behavior is occurring.

If you need to interview additional teachers or other adults (including parents), make copies of the first two pages of the F-BSP protocol and use the copies for as many interviews as you plan to conduct.

Step 2A: Propose a Testable Explanation

ABC Sequence

A testable explanation is one of the most important pieces of the F-BSP process. It is the summary of everything you have learned about the problem behavior and the link to designing an effective, relevant BSP.

Begin to build your testable hypothesis by listing the problem behavior. It is likely that a student will engage in more than one type of problem behavior. For example, the same student might fight with other students and refuse to follow teacher directions. List each *type* of problem behavior separately in the column labeled "Behavior." (Don't list every single problem behavior displayed. For example, if fighting consists of pushing, hitting, and yelling at other students, you would lump all three behaviors into one *type* of behavior: "fighting.")

Next, for each type of behavior you have listed, indicate the antecedents that tend to set off or predict that behavior. List them under the column headed "Antecedents." Refer back to the interview information to identify the antecedents.

For each type of behavior you have listed, indicate the consequences that tend to support the problem behavior in the "Consequences" column. The interviewee will have told you about many potential consequences that occur. List the ones that seem to make the behavior continue or worsen. For example, a student who makes inappropriate jokes in class might encounter two consequences. First, the joke might be ignored by other students, and he is unlikely to tell that joke again. Second, he might get a lot of attention and laughter over his inappropriate joke. In that case, he is likely to tell other inappropriate jokes or tell the same joke in other classes. In this example, the ignoring consequence did not support the problem behavior, but the attention/laughter consequence did. For your testable explanation of why the problem behavior is occurring, you want to list the consequences that support the problem behavior. In the example, you would write "peer attention and laughter" under the column that is headed "Consequences."

Finally, if there are any setting events that make the problem behavior worse or more likely to occur, list them under the column headed "Setting Event."

Complete the Setting Event, Antecedent, and Consequence boxes for each *type* of behavior that you have listed. Each set of these is called an *ABC sequence.*

Function of the Behavior

For each ABC sequence, you want to determine why you think the behavior is occurring. At this point you can describe the behavior, you know what situations set it off, and you know what consequences make it continue or get worse. But why is the behavior happening? What function does it serve for the student? Some common functions include: to get peer attention, to get adult attention, to get out of doing difficult work, or to get away from someone the student doesn't like. For each ABC sequence, decide what you think is really motivating the problem behavior and write it down in the space provided.

Once you become more familiar with the F-BSP Protocol, it will become fairly easy to complete Step 2. At that point, we suggest that you complete Step 2 with the interviewee to check for his or her agreement with your summary of the interview.

Functional Assessment Checklist
for Teachers and Staff (FACTS)

FACTS—PART A

Student/Grade: _____   **Date:** _____

Interviewer: _____   **Respondent(s):** _____

Student profile: Please identify at least three strengths or contributions the student brings to school.

_____

_____

Problem Behavior(s): Identify problem behaviors

___ Tardy	___ Inappropriate language	___ Disruptive	___ Theft
___ Unresponsive	___ Fight/physical aggression	___ Insubordination	___ Vandalism
___ Withdrawn	___ Verbal harassment	___ Work not done	___ Other_____

Describe problem behavior: _____

Identifying Routines: Where, when, and with whom problem behaviors are most likely.

Schedule (Times)	Activity	With Whom Does Problem Occur?	Likelihood of Problem Behavior	Specific Problem Behavior
			Low High 1 2 3 4 5 6	
			1 2 3 4 5 6	
			1 2 3 4 5 6	
			1 2 3 4 5 6	
			1 2 3 4 5 6	
			1 2 3 4 5 6	
			1 2 3 4 5 6	
			1 2 3 4 5 6	
			1 2 3 4 5 6	

Select one to three routines for further assessment. Select routines based on (1) similarity of activities (conditions) with ratings of 4, 5, or 6 and (2) similarity of problem behavior(s). Complete the FACTS–Part B for each routine identified.

(continued)

FACTS–Part B

Student/Grade: _____   Date: _____

Interviewer: _____   Respondent(s): _____

Routine/Activities/Context: Which routine (only one) from the FACTS–Part A is assessed?

Routine/Activities/Context	Problem Behavior

Provide more detail about the problem behavior(s):

What does the problem behavior(s) look like?
How often does the problem behavior(s) occur?
How long does the problem behavior(s) last when it does occur?
What is the intensity/level of danger of the problem behavior(s)?

What are the events that predict when the problem behavior(s) will occur?

Related Issues (Setting Events)		Environmental Features	
___ illness	Other: ___	___ reprimand/correction	___ structured activity
___ drug use	_____	___ physical demands	___ unstructured time
___ negative social	_____	___ socially isolated	___ tasks too boring
___ conflict at home	_____	___ with peers	___ activity too long
___ academic failure	_____	___ other	___ tasks too difficult

What consequences are most likely to maintain the problem behavior(s)?

Things That Are Obtained		Things Avoided or Escaped From	
___ adult attention	Other: _____	___ hard tasks	Other: _____
___ peer attention	_____	___ reprimands	_____
___ preferred activity	_____	___ peer negatives	_____
___ money/things	_____	___ physical effort	_____

SUMMARY OF BEHAVIOR

Identify the summary that will be used to build a plan of behavior support

Setting Events and Predictors	Problem Behavior(s)	Maintaining Consequence(s)

How confident are you that the Summary of Behavior is accurate?

Not very confident					Very confident
1	2	3	4	5	6

What current efforts have been used to control the problem behavior?

Strategies for Preventing Problem Behavior		Consequences for Problem Behavior	
___ schedule change	Other: _____	___ reprimand	Other: _____
___ seating change	_____	___ office referral	_____
___ curriculum change	_____	___ detention	_____

(continued)

Instructions

The FACTS is a two-page interview used by school personnel who are building behavior support plans. The FACTS is intended to be an efficient strategy for initial functional behavioral assessment. The FACTS is completed by people (teachers, family, clinicians) who know the student best, and is used to either build behavior support plans, or to guide more complete functional assessment efforts. The FACTS can be completed in a short period of time (5–15 minutes). Efficiency and effectiveness in completing the forms increases with practice.

How to Complete the FACTS–Part A

Step 1: Complete Demographic Information

Indicate the name and grade of the student, the date the assessment data were collected, the name of the person completing the form (the interviewer), and the name(s) of the people providing information (respondents).

Step 2: Complete Student Profile

Begin each assessment with a review of the positive and contributing characteristics the student brings to school. Identify at least three strengths or contributions the student offers.

Step 3: Identify Problem Behaviors

Identify the specific student behaviors that are barriers to effective education, disrupt the education of others, interfere with social development, or compromise safety at school. Provide a brief description of exactly how the student engages in these behaviors. What makes his or her way of doing these behaviors unique? Identify the most problematic behaviors, but also identify any problem behaviors that occur regularly.

Step 4: Identify Where, When, and with Whom the Problem Behaviors Are Most Likely

A: List the times that define the student's daily schedule. Include times between classes, lunch, and before school, and adapt for complex schedule features (e.g., odd/even days) if appropriate.

B: For each time listed indicate the activity typically engaged in during that time (e.g., small-group instruction, math, independent art, transition).

C: Where appropriate indicate the people (adults and peers) with whom the student is interacting during each activity, and especially list the people the student interacts with when he or she engages in problem behavior.

D: Use the 1 to 6 scale to indicate (in general) which times/activities are most and least likely to be associated with problem behaviors. A "1" indicates low likelihood of problems, and a "6" indicates high likelihood of problem behaviors.

E: Indicate which problem behavior is *most likely* in any time/activity that is given a rating of 4, 5, or 6.

Step 5: Select Routines for Further Assessment

Examine each time/activity listed as 4, 5, or 6 in the Table from Step 4. If activities are similar (e.g., activities that are unstructured; activities that involve high academic demands; activities with teacher reprimands; activities with peer taunting) and have similar problem behaviors, treat them as "routines for further analysis."

Select between one and three routines for further analysis. Write the name of the routine and the most common problem behavior(s). Within each routine identify the problem behavior(s) that are most likely or most problematic.

For *each* routine identified in Step 5 complete a FACTS–Part B.

(continued)

How to Complete the FACTS–Part B

Step 1: Complete Demographic Information

Identify the name and grade of the student, the date that the FACTS–Part B was completed, who completed the form, and who provided information for completing the form.

Step 2: Identify the Target Routine

List the targeted routine and problem behavior from the bottom of the FACTS–Part A. The FACTS–Part B provides information about *one* routine. Use multiple Part B forms if multiple routines are identified.

Step 3: Provide Specifics about the Problem Behavior(s)

Provide more detail about the features of the problem behavior(s). Focus specifically on the unique and distinguishing features, and the way the behavior(s) is disruptive or dangerous.

Step 4: Identify Events That Predict Occurrence of the Problem Behavior(s)

Within each routine what (1) setting events and (2) immediate preceding events predict when the problem behavior(s) will occur? What would you do to make the problem behaviors happen in this routine?

Step 5: Identify the Consequences That May Maintain the Problem Behavior

What consequences appear to reward the problem behavior? Consider that the student may get/obtain something he or she wants, or that he or she may escape/avoid something he or she finds unpleasant.

Identify the *most powerful* maintaining consequence with a "1," and other possible consequences with a "2" or "3." Do not check more than three options. The focus here is on the consequence that has the greatest impact.

When problems involve minor events that escalate into very difficult events, separate the consequences that maintain the minor problem behavior from the events that may maintain problem behavior later in the escalation.

Step 6: Define What Has Been Done to Date to Prevent/Control the Problem Behavior

In most cases, school personnel will have tried some strategies already. List events that have been tried, and organize these by (1) those things that have been done to prevent the problem from getting started, and (2) those things that were delivered as consequences to control or punish the problem behavior (or reward alternative behavior).

Step 7: Build a Summary Statement

The summary statement indicates the setting events, immediate predictors, problem behaviors, and maintaining consequences. The summary statement is the foundation for building an effective behavior support plan. Build the summary statement from the information in the FACTS–A and FACTS–B (especially the information in Steps 3, 4, and 5 of the FACTS–B). If you are confident that the summary statement is accurate enough to design a plan, move into plan development. If you are less confident, then continue the functional assessment by conducting direct observation.

References

Broussard, C., & Northup, J. (1997). The use of functional analysis to develop peer interventions for disruptive classroom behavior. *School Psychology Quarterly, 12*(11), 65–76.

Carr, E. G., Levin, L., McConnachie, G., Carlson, J. I., Kemp, D. C., Smith, C. E., & McLaughlin, D. M. (1999). Comprehensive multisituational intervention for problem behavior in the community: Long-term maintenance and social validation. *Journal of Positive Behavior Interventions, 1,* 5–25.

Colvin, G., Kameenui, E. J., & Sugai, G. (1993). School-wide and classroom management: Reconceptualizing the integration and management of students with behavior problems in general education. *Education and Treatment of Children, 16,* 361–381.

Crone, D. A., & Horner, R. H. (1999–2000). Contextual, conceptual, and empirical foundations of functional behavioral assessment in schools. *Exceptionality, 8*(3), 161–172.

Crone, D. A., & Horner, R. H. (2003). *Building positive behavior support systems in schools: Functional behavioral assessment.* New York: Guilford Press.

Davies, D. E., & McLaughlin, T. F. (1989). Effects of a daily report on disruptive behaviour in primary students. *BC Journal of Special Education, 13,* 173–181.

Didden, R., Duker, P. C., & Korzilius, H. (1997). Meta-analytic study on treatment effectiveness for problem behaviors with individuals who have mental retardation. *American Journal on Mental Retardation, 101,* 387–399.

Dougherty, E. H., & Dougherty, A. (1977). The daily report card: A simplified and flexible package for classroom behavior management. *Psychology in the Schools, 14*(2), 191–195.

Elliot, D. S., Hamburg, B. A., & Williams, K. R. (1998). *Violence in American schools: A new perspective.* New York: Cambridge University Press

Fairchild, T. N. (1987). The daily report card. *Teaching Exceptional Children, 19*(2), 72–73.

Fern Ridge Middle School, School Climate Committee Members, Fern Ridge School District 28J. (1999). *The High Five Program: A positive approach to school discipline.* Veneta, OR: Author.

Hawken, L. S. (2003). *The Behavior Education Program (BEP): Efficient and effective prevention of severe problem behavior in schools.* Manuscript submitted for publication.

Hawken, L. S., & Horner, R. H. (in press). Evaluation of a targeted intervention within a school-wide system of behavior support. *Journal of Behavioral Education.*

Horner, R. H., Albin, R. W., Sprague, J. R., & Todd, A. W. (1999). Positive behavior support. In M. E. Snell & F. Brown (Eds.), *Instruction of students with severe disabilities* (5th ed., pp. 207–243). Upper Saddle River, NJ: Merrill-Prentice-Hall.

Ingram, K. (2002). *Comparing effectiveness of intervention strategies that are based on functional behavioral assessment information and those that are contra-indicated by the assessment.* Unpublished dissertation, University of Oregon, Eugene.

Leach, D. J., & Byrne, M. K. (1986). Some "spill-over" effects of a home-based reinforcement programme in secondary school. *Educational Psychology, 6*(3), 265–276.

Lee, Y., Sugai, G., & Horner, R. (1999). Effect of component skill instruction on math performance and on-task, problem, and off-task behavior of students with emotional and behavioral disorders. *Journal of Positive Behavioral Interventions, 1,* 195–204.

Lewis, T. J., & Sugai, G. (1999). Effective behavior support: A systems approach to proactive school-wide management. *Effective School Practices, 17*(4), 47–53.

Lewis, T. J., Sugai, G., & Colvin, G. (1998). Reducing problem behavior through a school-wide system of effective behavioral support: Investigation of a school-wide social skills training program and contextual interventions. *School Psychology Review, 27,* 446–459.

Long, N., & Edwards, M. (1994). The use of a daily report card to address children's school behavior problems. *Contemporary Education, 65*(3), 152–155.

March, R., Lewis-Palmer, L., Brown, D., Crone, D., Todd, A. W., & Carr, E. (2000). *Functional assessment checklist for teachers and staff (FACTS).* Eugene: Educational and Community Supports, University of Oregon.

March, R. E., & Horner, R. H. (2002). Feasibility and contributions of functional behavioral assessment in schools. *Journal of Emotional and Behavioral Disorders, 10*(3), 158–170.

Nelson, J. R., Martella, R., & Galand, B. (1998). The effects of teaching school expectations and establishing consistent consequences on formal office disciplinary actions. *Journal of Emotional and Behavioral Disorders, 6*(3), 153–161.

Nelson, J. R., Martella, R. M., & Marchand-Martella, N. (2002). Maximizing student learning : The effects of a comprehensive school-based program for preventing problem behaviors. *Journal of Emotional and Behavioral Disorders, 10*(3), 136–148.

O'Neill, R. E., Horner, R. H., Albin, R. W., Sprague, J. R., Storey, K., & Newton, J. S. (1997). *Functional assessment for problem behavior: A practical handbook (2nd ed.).* Pacific Grove, CA: Brooks/Cole.

Sinclair, M. F., Christenson, S. L., Evelo, D. L., & Hurley, C. M. (1998). Dropout prevention for youth with disabilities: Efficacy of a sustained school engagement procedure. *Exceptional Children, 65*(1), 7–21.

Sprague, J., Walker, H., Golly, A., White, K., Meyers, D., & Shannon, T. (2001). Translating research into effective practice: The effects of a universal staff and student intervention on indicators of discipline and school safety. *Education and Treatment of Children, 24*(4), 495–511.

Sugai, G., & Horner, R. H. (1999). Discipline and behavioral support: Preferred processes and practices. *Effective School Practices, 17*(4), 10–22.

Sugai, G., & Horner, R. H. (2002). The evolution of discipline practices: School-wide positive behavior supports. *Child and Family Behavior Therapy.*

Sugai, G., Horner, R. H., Dunlap, G., Hieneman, M., Lewis, T. J., Nelson, C. M., Scott, T., Liaupsin, C., Sailor, W., Turnbull, A. P., Turnbull, H. R., III, Wickham, D., Wilcox, B., & Ruef, M. (2000). Applying positive behavior support and functional behavioral assessment in schools. *Journal of Positive Behavior Interventions, 2*(3), 131–143.

Sugai, G., Lewis-Palmer, T., & Hagan-Burke, S. (1999–2000). Overview of the functional assessment process. *Exceptionality, 8*(3), 149–160.

Taylor-Greene, S., Brown, D., Nelson, L., Longton, J., Gassman, T., Cohen, J., Swartz, J., Horner, R. H., Sugai, G., & Hall, S. (1997). School-wide behavioral support: Starting the year off right. *Journal of Behavioral Education, 7,* 99–112.

Todd, A. W., Horner, R. H., Sugai, G., & Colvin, G. (1999). Individualizing school-wide discipline for students with chronic problem behaviors: A team approach. *Effective School Practices, 17*(4), 72–82.

Tyack, D. (2001). Introduction. In S. Mondale & S. Patton (Eds.), *School: The story of American Public Education.* Boston: Beacon Press.

U.S. Department of Health and Human Services. (2001). *Youth violence: A report of the Surgeon General.* Washington, DC: Office of the Surgeon General.

Vollmer, T. R., & Northrup, J. (1996). Some implications of functional analysis for school psychology. *School Psychology Quarterly, 11,* 76–92.

Walker, H. M., Horner, R. H., Sugai, G., Bullis, M., Sprague, J. R., Bricker, D., & Kaufman, M. J. (1996). Integrated approaches to preventing antisocial behavior patterns among school-age children and youth. *Journal of Emotional and Behavioral Disorders, 4,* 194–209.

Warberg, A., George, N., Brown, D., Chauran, K., & Taylor-Greene, S. (1995). *Behavior Education Plan Handbook.* Elmira, OR: Fern Ridge Middle School.

Index

i indicates an illustration; *t* indicates a table.